Epidemiology and Non-Drug Treatment of Head Pain

Research and Clinical Studies in Headache

Vol. 5

Series Editors
A. P. FRIEDMAN, Tucson, Ariz., and MARY E. GRANGER, North Caldwell, N.J.

Editorial Board
M. CRITCHELEY, London; J.M. ESPADALER, Barcelona; S.H. FRAZIER, New York, N.Y.; J.R. GRAHAM, Boston, Mass.; P. KALLOS, Helsingborg; J.W. LANCE, Sydney; R.J.L. PLUVINAGE, Paris; G.F. POCH, Buenos Aires; H. ROME, Rochester, Minn.; SICUTERI, Florence

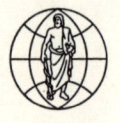

S. Karger · Basel · München · Paris · London · New York · Sydney

Epidemiology and Non-Drug Treatment of Head Pain

Volume Editor
Mary E. Granger, North Caldwell, N. J.

17 figures and 18 tables, 1978

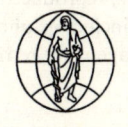

S. Karger · Basel · München · Paris · London · New York · Sydney

Research and Clinical Studies in Headache
An International Review

Vol. 1: X + 221 p., 69 fig., 17 tab., 1967
ISBN 3-8055-0616-3
Vol. 2: VIII + 225 p., 25 fig., 17 tab., 1969
ISBN 3-8055-0617-1
Vol. 3: X + 380 p., 191 fig., 51 tab., 1972
ISBN 3-8055-1295-3
Vol. 4: Pathophysiologic, Diagnostic and Therapeutic Aspects of Headache.
Eds. M.E. Granger (North Caldwell, N.J.) and G. Poch (Buenos Aires).
VIII + 128 p., 20 fig., 12 tab., 1976
ISBN 3-8055-2282-7

Cataloging in Publication
Epidemiology and non-drug treatment of head pain
Volume editor, Mary E. Granger. – Basel, New York, Karger, 1978.
(Research and clinical studies in headache, vol. 5)
1. Headache – occurrence 2. Headache – therapy 3. Physical Therapy
I. Granger, Mary E., ed. II. Title III. Series
W1 RE215B v. 5/WL 342 E64
ISBN 3-8055-2803-5

All rights reserved.
No part of this publication may be translated into other languages, reproduced or utilized in any form or by any means, electronic or mechanical, including photocopying, recording, microcopying, or by any information storage and retrieval system, without permission in writing from the publisher.

© Copyright 1978 by S. Karger AG, 4101 Basel (Switzerland), Arnold-Böcklin-Strasse 25
Printed in Switzerland by Gasser & Cie AG, Basel
ISBN 3-8055-2803-5

Contents

Preface IX

Epidemiological Aspects of Headache

A Survey of Headache in an English City
C. A. Newland, L. S. Illis, P. K. Robinson, B. G. Batchelor and W. E. Waters (Southampton) 1

The Background 1
Prevalence 2
Definition 2
Validation 3
The Southampton Survey 5
Survey Method 5
Response 7
The Sample 7
Results 9
Discussion 16
Acknowledgements 20
References 20

The Epidemiology and Genetics of Migraine
D. K. Ziegler (Kansas City, Kans.) 21

Migraine in Childhood
C. F. Barlow (Boston, Mass.) 34

Introduction 34
Substrate of Childhood Migraine 36

Expression of Childhood Migraine 37
    Common Migraine 37
    Classic Migraine 37
    Cyclic Vomiting 37
    Abdominal Migraine 38
    Convulsions Associated with Migraine 38
    Ophthalmoplegic Migraine 38
    Hemiplegic Migraine, including Aphasia and Focal Somatic Sensory
      Phenomena 39
    Basilar Artery Migraine 39
    Confusional States 40
Benign Paroxysmal Vertigo 40
Paroxysmal Leg Pain 41
Psychogenic Headaches 41
Symptomatic Vascular Headaches – Differential Diagnosis and Ancillary Studies ... 41
Treatment 43
Prognosis 44
References 45

Non-Drug Treatments of Head Pain

Autogenic Biofeedback Treatment for Migraine
S.L. Fahrion (Rochester) 47

Introduction 47
Autogenic Biofeedback Training 48
Single Group Outcome Studies 50
Controlled Studies 56
Possible Mechanisms 59
Training Procedures 63
Conclusions 68
References 69

Acupuncture in Headache
J.J. Bischko (Vienna) 72

Cryosurgery of Headache
N. Cook (Victoria, B.C.) 86

Introduction 86
Development of Procedure 87
Rationale 87
Indications 88

Contents

Contraindications	88
Results	88
Anatomic and other Considerations	90
Surgery	91
Phenomena Observed during Cryosurgery in the Sphenopalatine Area	94
Animal Experiments	96
The Transantral Approach	99
Complications	99
Postoperative Course	100
Summary	101
References	101

Stereotactic Treatment of Head and Neck Pain
  P.L. GILDENBERG (Houston, Tex.) 102

Introduction	102
Human Stereotactic Surgery	103
Stereotactic Procedures for Treatment of Pain	104
Stimulation Produced Analgesia	107
Clinical Indications	110
Cancer Pain	110
Thalamic Syndrome	112
Trigeminal Neuralgia	113
Anesthesia Dolorosa	114
Postherpetic Neuralgia	115
Atypical Facial Neuralgia	115
Headache	115
References	116

Chronic Brain Stimulation for the Treatment of Intractable Pain
  Y. HOSOBUCHI (San Francisco, Calif.) 122

Preface

As readers are well aware, headache is a symptom and it is necessary to consider not just the treatment of the symptom but of the whole patient. In the first article in Volume 1 of this series, E. C. KUNKLE quoted Plato's advice: '... for the part can never be well unless the whole is well; let no one persuade you to cure the head until he has first given you his soul to be cured.'

One of the purposes of this series on *Research and Clinical Studies in Headache* is to draw attention to various advances in techniques in research, diagnosis and treatment which will better help the clinican treat the 'whole patient'.

Whereas there have been recent pharmacological and psychological advances in the field of headache research, the current volume covers two other general areas. It is arbitrarily divided into two parts: the first, 'Epidemiological Aspects of Headache', and the second, 'Non-drug Treatments of Head Pain'. A brief explanation of the nature of the papers in each section and the reason for their selection is appropriate.

Of the three papers in Part I, 'A Survey of Headache in an English City' is strictly epidemiological. 'The Epidemiology and Genetics of Migraine', as the title indicates, also deals with the genetics of migraine. 'Migraine in Childhood', while a comprehensive discussion of that subject, is included in this section because of its epidemiological emphasis.

The non-drug treatment of head pain is almost open-ended in its scope. It will be evident that not all non-drug treatments of head pain can be included in Part II of this volume. Psychotherapy and allergic management are obvious omissions of orthodox treatment while transcendental meditation, sleep therapy and yoga are less orthodox treatments which have not been included.

Preface

The five papers contained in Part II have been selected for their interest and challenge, but not on the basis that the treatment they describe is advocated by the editors. The papers on autogenic biofeedback and acupuncture are included because of the recent, increased medical and public interest these methods have attracted. While neurosurgical intervention for the alleviation of head pain is a last resort, it may indeed be necessary in cases intractable to all other forms of treatment. Part II contains three papers describing neurosurgical procedures for pain relief in such problem cases and the results of such treatment. Although the paper by HOSOBUCHI deals with the neurosurgical approach to the broader topic of intractable pain of CNS or peripheral origin, his use of brain stimulation for pain control offers a 'nondestructive, nonaddictive means of alleviating chronic pain', which can also be applied to chronic head pain.

ARNOLD P. FRIEDMAN
MARY E. GRANGER

A Survey of Headache in an English City

C. A. Newland, L. S. Illis, P. K. Robinson, B. G. Batchelor and W. E. Waters

Departments of Community Medicine and Electronics, University of Southampton and Wessex Neurological Centre, Southampton General Hospital, Southampton

Contents

The Background	1
Prevalence	2
Definition	2
Validation	3
The Southampton Survey	5
Survey Method	5
Response	7
The Sample	7
Results	9
Discussion	16
Acknowledgements	20
References	20

The Background

Headache is one of the most common of all symptoms and has a recorded history dating back several thousand years. Very few people have never experienced a headache and yet, surprisingly, there has been little research until recently on the epidemiology of this symptom. Headache and migraine are common phenomena in many countries of the world. Perhaps because they do not kill, or are not permanently disabling, they do not attract much research attention. However, severe headache and migraine can be very disruptive to social and family life as well as accounting for considerable time lost from work. In Britain in 1968/69, 295,000 man days and 167,000 woman days were lost because of migraine [Office of Health

Economics, 1972]. These figures are derived from sickness absence certification statistics and are therefore a considerable underestimate as certification is only made in cases of absence for 3 days or more, and few migraine attacks last this long. It is likely that the majority of headache and migraine attacks result in a maximum of one day's work loss. In addition to the large cost to the nation in terms of sickness absence in 1970 the cost of migraine to the National Health Service was a minimum of £ 2.8 million [Office of Health Economics, 1972]. Again, this figure is known to be an underestimate as it excludes significant outpatient expenditure on migraine for which there is no specific data. It is also known that a large number of people do not consult their doctor because they believe that the doctor cannot do anything for them anyway or because they believe in self-medication. Official statistics therefore can only hint at the size of the problem. In the absence of any reliable statistics it is left for the research worker to discover the prevalence of the condition and to do this it is necessary to organise research specifically for this purpose.

Prevalence

A number of studies have attempted to determine the prevalence of migraine. The figures produced vary considerably. For instance, FITZ-HUGH [1940] in a study of patients produced a prevalence rate as high as 200 per 1,000 population while BREWIS *et al.* [1966] using general practitioners' lists, produced a prevalence figure of only 5 per 1,000 population. There are many reasons for large discrepancies in figures between different researchers. One possible reason could be the use of different sampling frames. Research has been done in such groups as school children [BILLE, 1962], doctors [DALSGAARD-NIELSON and ULRICH, 1973], prisoners [WATERS, 1974a] and factory workers [CHILDS and SWEETNAM, 1961], all producing rather different prevalence figures. However, perhaps the main reason for such variance is the wide difference of opinion as to what constitutes migraine.

Definition

The problems of defining migraine can quickly be recognised by a glance at any neurology textbook. Any definition given allows plenty of scope for interpretation. Any one definition may mention some or all of a wide variety of symptoms. The most commonly mentioned symptoms are headache and nausea. The headache of migraine is typically described as a throbbing pain on one side of the head, usually the temple, but headache in many different forms and degrees of intensity may also be associated with migraine. Similarly, nausea might mean anything from persistent violent attacks associated with vomiting to an intermittent feeling of slight sickness. Other typical symptoms are numerous although, again, they need not always be present in an attack. They include visual disturbance, feelings of dizziness, sensations of heat, abdominal pain and changes in mood, to name but a few.

In view of the large divergence of opinion as to what actually constitutes a migraine attack the World Federation of Neurology's Research Group on Migraine and Headache [1969] attempted to define the condition. The definition they eventually produced was as follows: 'Recurrent attacks of headache, widely varied in intensity, frequency and duration. The attacks are commonly unilateral in onset; are usually associated with anorexia and, sometimes, with nausea and vomiting; in some are preceded by, or associated with, conspicuous sensory, motor, and mood disturbances; and are often familial.'

As is the case with other definitions it fails to specify clear-cut criteria on which diagnosis may be based. There are no clinical tests to establish diagnosis, so the researcher is left to establish his own criteria. These criteria may, or may not, coincide with the concensus of clinical opinion and the only way of finding out is to compare the researcher's 'on paper' diagnosis with a clinical assessment.

Validation

In view of the considerable difficulties in defining migraine, a series of studies in Wales [WATERS, 1970, 1971; WATERS and O'CONNOR, 1971] attempted to tackle the problem in a rather different manner. In these surveys, members of the public were selected at random from the electoral roll and asked to complete a questionnaire concerning their headaches, if any. No attempt was made to define migraine in the questionnaire and the word 'migraine' was deliberately not mentioned. However, the questionnaire did ask for details about any headaches which had occurred in the previous year and about the typical symptoms of a migraine attack. It was then possible to calculate the prevalence of headache and the prevalence of some of the typical migraine symptoms.

Having done this, the questionnaire findings were compared with a neurologist's clinical diagnosis on the same individuals. This clinical validation of the questionnaire was confined to the *women* in the sample. It showed clearly that there were three important features which, above all else, influenced the diagnosis of migraine. These were the presence or absence of the following: (1) a unilateral distribution of headache; (2) a warning that the headache was coming, and (3) nausea or vomiting accompanying the headache.

---

13. Are your headaches one side only?
    never? ......
    sometimes? ...... Please tick one ▢ 28.
    usually? ......
    always? ......

14. *Before you get a headache* do you know that one is coming?
    never? ......
    sometimes? ...... Please tick one ▢ 29.
    usually? ......
    always? ......

    If you do, please tick any groups that apply

    (a) changes in mood (elation, depression), increased energy ...... ▢ 30.

    (b) watery eyes, dislike of light, blurred vision, double vision, dimness of vision ...... ▢ 31.

    (c) zigzag flashes of light, coloured lights ...... ▢ 32.

    (d) blind areas in field of vision ...... ▢ 33.

    (e) pins and needles ...... ▢ 34.

    (f) feeling of sickness ...... ▢ 35.

    (g) other ...... ▢ 36.

    If other, please give details

17. *When you have a headache* do you
    ever feel sick? ......
    usually feel sick? ...... Please tick all
    ever vomit? ...... that apply ▢ 43.
    usually vomit? ...... ▢ 44.

Fig. 1. Questions used in the Southampton survey to determine the three features of migraine: unilateral distribution, warning and nausea.

Figure 1 shows the questions designed to elicit this information, as they appeared on the questionnaire.

Migraine was diagnosed clinically in 87.5% of women in whom all three features were present; in between 31.8 and 60.0% if only two features (depending on which two) were present; and in between 11.8 and 50.0% if only one feature was present. It was therefore possible to use these figures to calculate a prevalence rate for migraine in the previous year and this was estimated at 19% for the women aged 20–64 years [WATERS and O'CONNOR, 1971]. The questionnaire used in the surveys in Wales was thus validated by clinical assessment for women. As the diagnosis of migraine is based on symptoms, it seems fair to assume that the questionnaire used will be equally valid for men. This hypothesis is currently being tested in Southampton with data from the headache survey which took place between July 1973 and February 1974.

The Southampton Survey

Previous surveys have shown that many sufferers of moderately severe headache and migraine do not attend a doctor [WATERS, 1974a]. It is likely, therefore, that a study of headache and migraine in the general population will lead to more accurate knowledge of the aetiology of these conditions. As the diagnosis of migraine is almost entirely dependent on symptoms, it should be possible to use a self-administered questionnaire to elicit a history of the symptoms on which diagnosis depends. In the Southampton survey, the questionnaire previously validated (for women) in South Wales was used as a basis for the survey, but some questions were altered and new questions were added. The Southampton survey therefore built on earlier work. It attempted to improve the quality of information collected and it is being followed by a validation of the questions by two neurologists. This validation is being completed in both men and women and techniques of pattern recognition are being applied to the data.

Survey Method

Southampton is a growing city with a population of over 200,000 inhabitants. As well as being a major European port, it has a variety of industry and a growing University. The city covers an area which is approximately

7 miles from East to West and 4 miles from North to South. As it was envisaged that some of the survey sample would need to be visited at home in order to secure a high response rate, it was decided to restrict the survey area to a defined geographical area of the city. It was hoped that the chosen area would provide a reasonable cross section of the population with regard to social class. The survey area was thus delineated after careful consideration of the available statistics on social class [Office of Population, Censuses and Surveys, 1966]. The area chosen covered seven electoral wards of the Southampton Test Parliamentary Constituency. The General Hospital, where the research project was based, was near the centre of this area which encompassed a wide variety of land use from docklands to an expensive residential area neighbouring the University. The current register of electors for the area was then obtained. This had been published in February 1973 although the qualifying date had, in fact, been somewhat earlier in October 1972. It was then calculated that in order to achieve the required sample size a sampling interval of 20 was required. Every 20th name was then chosen for the sample, except where it was indicated that the person so chosen was a merchant seamen, service voter or youth. It was thought that the merchant seaman and service voters might prove difficult to contact and that the youths, those not yet 18 but who would have their 18th birthday during the currency of the electoral roll, would be unrepresentative of all 17 year olds. Altogether 57 people were thus excluded leaving a final survey sample of 2,508.

Questionnaires were then despatched area by area. It was considered essential to attain a high response rate and, having studied the literature on mail survey method (particularly SCOTT [1961]), it was decided that the most practical way of attempting to do so was to use two reminders. These were to be sent 2 and 6 weeks after the initial approach. It was also decided that those who did not respond to these three requests would be visited at their homes. At both the initial approach and the two follow-ups a copy of the questionnaire was accompanied by a covering letter and a pre-paid envelope for reply. In this way a response rate of 84.5% was achieved by post which was increased to 89.4% after an interviewer had visited non-respondents at home.

The whole questionnaire was 7 pages long and was divided into three sections of questions. The first section, covering less than a page, asked for general information such as age, sex, marital status and occupation. The next asked for details of headaches experienced in the past year including questions on duration, severity and accompanying symptoms. Next followed

Table I. Survey response

	n	%
Questionnaires sent	2,508	
Exclusions		
Left area	168	
Dead	29	
Total	197	
Resultant survey population	2,311	100
Completed questionnaires	2,066	89.4
Refusals	110	4.8
Uncontacted	98	4.2
Aged or ill	37	1.6

two pages of short questions from the Cornell Medical Index from which it was possible to calculate a 'neurotic score' for each respondent. The questionnaire concluded with a space left free for any comments.

Response

Questionnaires were sent to a total of 2,508 individuals. Subsequently it was discovered that 29 of these had died and a further 168 had left the survey area. Both of these groups were therefore excluded. It was not possible to contact 98 of the remaining sample despite at least two visits to each address. A further 110 refused to co-operate in the survey, either in writing or when the interviewer called. Finally, a small group of 37 people were excluded on the grounds of illness and/or old age. Completed questionnaires were therefore eventually received from 2,066 individuals who represented 89.4% of the eligible sample (table I).

The Sample

A comparison of the age and sex distribution of the survey population with that of the population of England and Wales [Office of Population, Censuses and Surveys, 1975] showed that women were slightly over-represented. Women made up 54.5% of the survey population, whereas the percentage of females in the population over 18 years old is 52.4%.

Figure 2 shows a comparison of the sample population with the general population by age group. It shows that in the age group 55–74 for both sexes the sample population is over-represented. This is compensated for by slight deficiencies in all the younger age groups. A possible reason for the deficiencies in the younger groups might well be their greater mobility.

Another comparison was made with the general population in respect of social class. The details given regarding occupation were used to classify

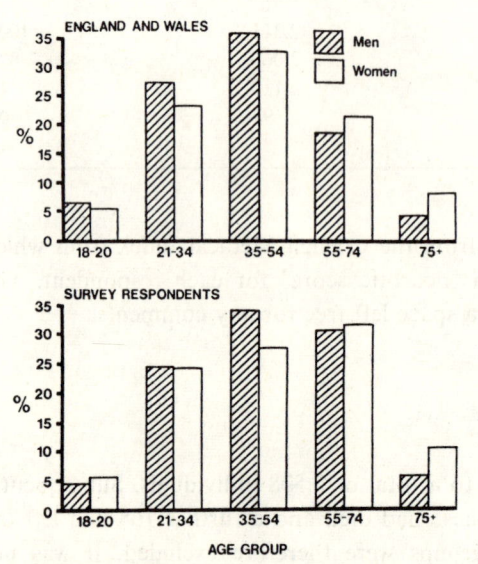

Fig. 2. Comparison of survey respondents with population of England and Wales, by age and sex.

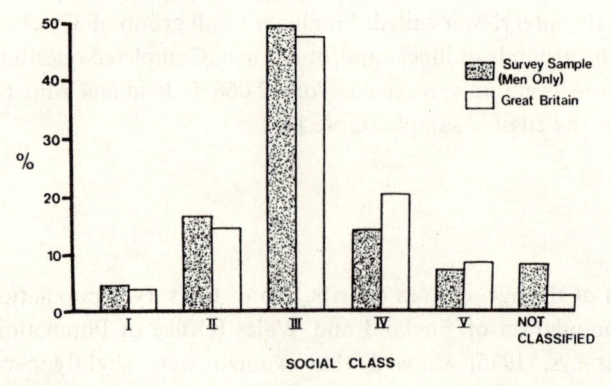

Fig. 3. Comparison of male survey respondents with population of Great Britain, by social class.

each person on the Registrar General's I–V scale of social class [Office of Population, Censuses and Surveys, 1970]. Although this exercise was completed for both men and women, it was thought that the information was unreliable for women due to their tendency to misinterpret the question and record their own rather than their husband's occupation as requested. The social class breakdown of respondents is therefore given for men only (fig. 3). Social classes I and II (the professional groups) were slightly over-represented. As it happened the social class III group was also slightly over-represented with a consequent deficiency in groups IV and V. The high percentage of unclassified occupations was due to insufficient details of occupation being recorded. In summary, the survey respondents were fairly representative of the general population but had a slightly higher proportion of women and of the higher social classes and more were in the age group 55–74 than expected.

Results[1]

The prevalence of headache in the previous year is given in table II. It shows that 73.1% of the men and 81.4% of the women had headache in the previous year, and that in all age groups more women had headaches than men. For both sexes there was a decline in prevalence with increasing age. Of those with headache 28% of the men and 41% of the women had consulted a doctor at some time in their lives because of headache, but only 12% of the men with headache and 19% of the women with headache had consulted a doctor in the year immediately preceding the survey. Although headache is less prevalent in the over 75-year age group the proportion with this symptom who consulted a doctor was high in both sexes (table III).

Although most of the questionnaire was designed to elicit information about the most severe headaches which each individual had experienced in the previous year, one question asked which headaches were usually experienced: mild only, severe only or both mild and severe. The results showed that 50% of those with headache in the previous year had mild headache only, 5% severe only and 45% both mild and severe. In all age groups women had both mild and severe headaches more frequently than men.

Severity of headache was recorded on a six point graded scale ranging from 'My headaches are very mild' (1) to 'My headaches are almost unbearable' (6). The distribution of headache severity showed no important

[1] For the analysis of each individual question the totals do not always reach 100% due to some individuals omitting certain questions, or giving an unclassifiable response.

Table II. Headache in previous year by age and sex (percentage in brackets)

	Men						Women					
	age, years					total	age, years					total
	18–20	21–34	35–54	55–74	75+		18–20	21–	35–54	55–74	75+	
Headache	40 (87.0)	205 (88.0)	257 (80.3)	159 (56.0)	25 (45.5)	686 (73.1)	59 (93.7)	267 (96.7)	286 (91.1)	247 (68.0)	58 (52.7)	917 (81.4)
No headache	6 (13.0)	28 (12.0)	63 (19.7)	125 (44.0)	30 (54.5)	253 (26.9)	4 (6.3)	9 (3.3)	28 (8.9)	116 (32.0)	52 (47.3)	209 (18.6)
Total	46 (100)	233 (100)	320 (100)	284 (100)	55 (100)	939 (100)	63 (100)	276 (100)	314 (100)	363 (100)	110 (100)	1,126 (100)

Table III. Distribution of subjects with headache in the previous year who had consulted a doctor about their headaches by age and sex (percentage of those with headache in brackets)

	Men						Women					
	age, years					total	age, years					total
	18–	21–	35–	55–	75–		18–	21–	35–	55–	75–	
Doctor never consulted	30 (75.0)	155 (75.6)	183 (71.2)	115 (72.3)	14 (56.0)	497 (72.4)	44 (74.6)	156 (58.4)	176 (61.5)	144 (58.3)	28 (48.3)	548 (59.8)
Doctor consulted but not in previous year	3 (7.5)	32 (15.6)	40 (15.6)	29 (18.2)	3 (12.0)	107 (15.6)	12 (20.3)	59 (22.1)	60 (21.0)	57 (23.1)	11 (19.0)	199 (21.7)
Doctor consulted in previous year	7 (17.5)	18 (8.8)	34 (13.2)	15 (9.4)	8 (32.0)	82 (12.0)	3 (5.1)	52 (19.5)	50 (17.5)	46 (18.6)	19 (32.7)	170 (18.5)

A Survey of Headache in an English City

Table IV. Severity of headache in previous year by age and sex (percentage of those with headache in brackets)

Severity	Men age, years						Women age, years					
	18–	21–	35–	55–	75–	total	18–	21–	35–	55–	75–	total
1 Very mild	6 (15)	24 (12)	41 (16)	39 (25)	7 (30)	117 (17.1)	6 (10)	21 (8)	32 (11)	45 (18)	19 (33)	123 (13.4)
2 Mild	20 (49)	67 (33)	80 (31)	50 (32)	10 (43)	227 (33.1)	15 (25)	56 (21)	54 (19)	70 (28)	17 (29)	212 (23.1)
3 Not usually severe	7 (17)	51 (25)	58 (22)	41 (26)	2 (9)	159 (23.2)	15 (25)	54 (20)	79 (28)	66 (27)	8 (14)	222 (24.2)
4 Quite severe	5 (12)	42 (20)	50 (19)	21 (13)	4 (17)	122 (17.8)	19 (32)	87 (33)	72 (25)	45 (18)	12 (21)	235 (25.6)
5 Very severe	3 (7)	12 (6)	14 (5)	4 (3)	0 (0)	33 (4.8)	2 (3)	32 (12)	31 (11)	14 (6)	2 (3)	81 (8.8)
6 Almost unbearable	0 (0)	9 (4)	16 (6)	3 (2)	0 (0)	28 (4.1)	2 (3)	17 (6)	18 (6)	9 (4)	0 (0)	46 (5.0)

Table V. Three features of migraine in previous year in relation to severity of headache (percentage of those with headache in brackets)

	Men severity						total	Women severity						total
	1	2	3	4	5	6		1	2	3	4	5	6	
Number with unilateral distribution	26 (24)	78 (35)	82 (53)	56 (46)	18 (55)	18 (64)	278 (41)	40 (35)	80 (38)	132 (59)	144 (61)	56 (69)	31 (67)	483 (53)
Number with warning	31 (28)	82 (37)	87 (56)	84 (69)	25 (76)	24 (86)	333 (49)	40 (35)	92 (45)	156 (70)	175 (74)	64 (79)	38 (83)	565 (63)
Number with nausea	14 (13)	53 (24)	53 (34)	59 (48)	22 (67)	21 (75)	222 (33)	15 (13)	60 (29)	105 (47)	143 (61)	61 (75)	40 (87)	424 (47)

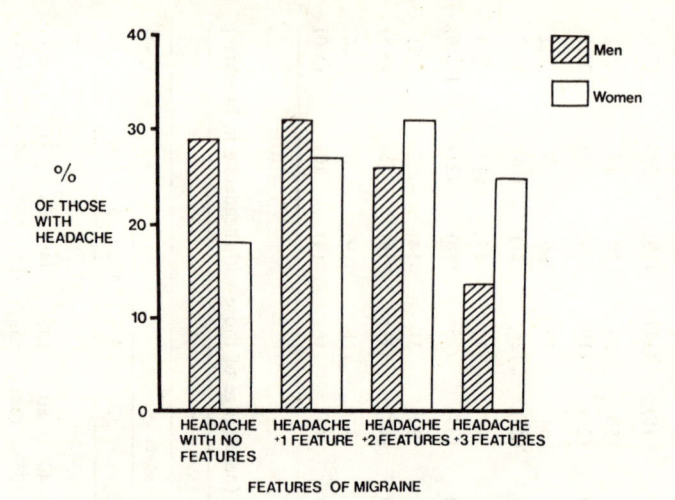

Fig. 4. Distribution of three features of migraine (unilateral distribution, warning and nausea) by sex.

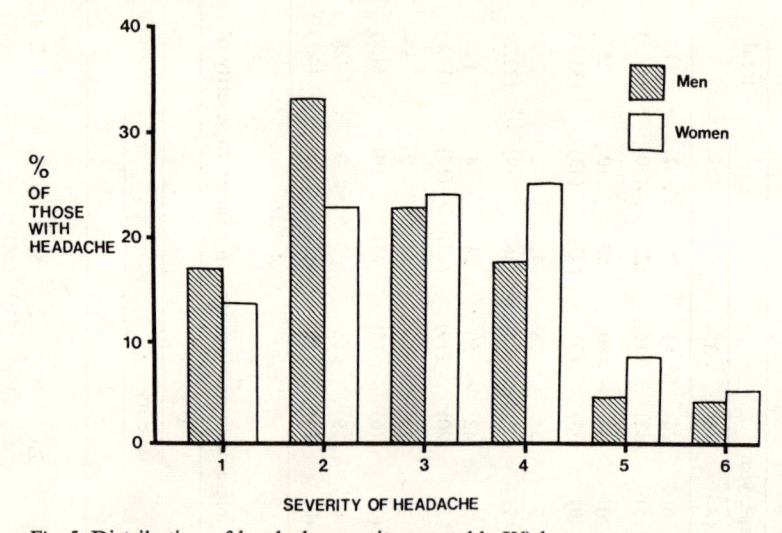

Fig. 5. Distribution of headache severity (see table IV) by sex.

differences with age, but on the whole more women reported severe headache than men (table IV, fig. 5). The proportion of subjects having three features of migraine – a unilateral distribution, a warning that the headache was coming and accompanying nausea (fig. 1) was related to severity of headache. Each of the three features became significantly more common as severity increased (table V). This was especially so in the case of nausea (fig. 6).

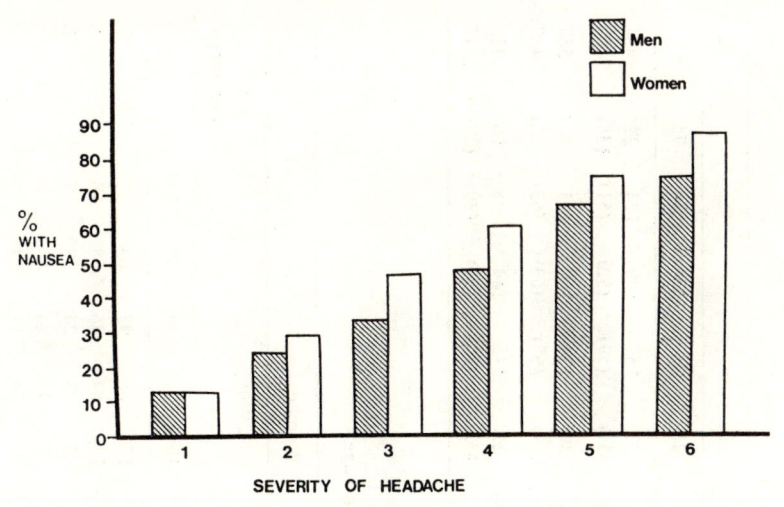

Fig. 6. Distribution of nausea by headache severity (see table IV).

Figure 4 shows the distribution of migrainous features by sex. It shows that women are more likely to have headaches with 2 or 3 migrainous features than men.

Table VI shows the distribution of the three individual features of migraine by age and sex. The percentage who had a unilateral distribution of headache – sometimes, usually or always – was 41 in men and 53 in women. There was a warning that the headache was coming for 49% of men and 62% of women with headache.

The nature of the warning symptoms was very similar for men and women (table VII). The most common for both men and women were changes in mood and sickness and the least common was pins and needles.

The third migrainous feature, nausea, was recorded for 33% of men with headache and 47% of women (tableVI). However, only 5% of men and 10% of women with headache had actually vomited during a headache attack in the previous year.

Another symptom associated with migraine is the presence of visual symptoms accompanying the headache. Some sort of visual symptom was present in 38% of men and 53% of women during a headache. The most common visual symptom was a minor disturbance such as watery eyes. Disturbances more commonly associated with migraine such as zigzag flashes of light and blind spots in the field of vision were experienced by 12% of men and 16% of women with headache (table VIII). Paraesthesia accompanied headache in 5% of men and 5% of women with headache.

Table VI. Three features of migraine in those with headache in previous year by age and sex (percentage of those with headache in brackets)

	Men						Women					
	age, years					total	age, years					total
	18–	21–	35–	55–	75–		18–	21–	35–	55–	75–	
Number with unilateral distribution	15 (37)	86 (42)	111 (43)	63 (41)	5 (22)	280 (41)	32 (54)	157 (59)	149 (52)	124 (51)	22 (38)	484 (53)
Number with warning	20 (50)	104 (51)	118 (46)	79 (51)	14 (61)	335 (49)	30 (51)	174 (65)	180 (63)	153 (63)	30 (52)	567 (62)
Number with nausea	10 (25)	75 (37)	100 (39)	31 (20)	7 (30)	223 (33)	25 (42)	145 (55)	144 (51)	95 (39)	16 (28)	425 (47)

Table VII. Nature of warning that a headache is coming, in the previous year, by sex and age

Warning[1] (selected from given list, see fig. 1)	Men							Women						
	age, years					total warnings		age, years					total warnings	
	18–	21–	35–	55–	75–	n	%	18–	21–	35–	55–	75–	n	%
Changes in mood	14	47	53	35	3	152	29	17	86	93	63	6	265	27
Watery eyes	6	38	45	32	8	129	24	14	84	56	58	18	230	24
Zigzag flashes	1	10	21	15	1	48	9	3	23	24	38	7	95	10
Blind areas	2	8	21	16	2	49	9	2	13	24	15	6	60	6
Pins and needles	0	7	8	8	1	24	5	0	14	13	24	2	53	5
Sickness	7	36	64	20	3	130	24	11	87	96	63	9	266	28

[1] Not mutually exclusive.

Table VIII. Subjects with visual symptoms during headaches in the previous year (percentage of those with headache)

Visual symptoms[1]	Men		Women	
	n	%	n	%
Watery eyes, etc.	213	31	367	40
Zigzag flashes, etc.	55	8	101	11
Blind areas, etc.	31	4	47	5
Other visual symptoms	16	2	32	4

[1] Not mutually exclusive.

Table IX. Distribution of subjects whose headaches are usually or always throbbing by pattern of headache in the previous year

Pattern	Men	Women
Headache only		
Number in group	198	160
Number throbbing	29	23
%	15	14
Headache + 1 feature		
Number in group	212	247
Number throbbing	43	66
%	20	27
Headache + 2 features		
Number in group	178	280
Number throbbing	51	108
%	29	39
Headache + 3 features		
Number in group	90	223
Number throbbing	44	128
%	49	57

The proportion of subjects who stated that their severe headaches are usually or always throbbing was related to the pattern of their headaches (table IX). For example, 49% of men with headache and the three features, but only 15% with headache and no migraine features, said that their headaches were usually or always throbbing; the equivalent figures for women were 57 and 14%. Overall, 25% of men and 36% of women had headaches that were usually or always throbbing. In addition, 48.5% of

Table X. Association of three features of migraine with each other (percentage in brackets)

Feature	Men					Women				
	number of persons	number with				number of persons	number with			
		unilateral distribution	warning	nausea	neither		unilateral distribution	warning	nausea	neither
Unilateral distribution	278 (100)		176 (63)	111 (40)	83 (30)	483 (100)		338 (70)	260 (54)	109 (23)
warning	333 (100)	176 (53)		161 (48)	88 (26)	565 (100)	338 (60)		351 (62)	101 (18)
Nausea	222 (100)	111 (50)	161 (73)		41 (18)	424 (100)	260 (61)	351 (83)		37 (9)

men and 43.3% of women with headache had throbbing headaches on some occasions only.

Table X shows how the three principal features of migraine are associated with each other. Of the three features nausea seems to be the least likely and unilateral distribution the most likely to be the only feature present. There was no association between the number of features present and social class.

In attempting to discover the amount of sickness absence due to headache the men were asked if they had missed work because of headache in the previous year and, if so, on how many days. Unfortunately many answers were unspecific stating, for instance, that 'several' or 'many' days had been missed. However, we were able to calculate that a minimum of 154 working days had been lost in the previous year due to headache in the total group of 939 men aged over 18 years. The number of days lost increased directly with the number of features of migraine present (table XI).

Discussion

The results of this survey in a defined area of the city of Southampton are in general similar to other community studies, for example the 1968 survey in the Pontypridd area in Wales [WATERS, 1974b]. The prevalence of headache in the various age groups was similar. Headaches were more common in women than in men and in both sexes declined with age. The

Table XI. Distribution of men aged 18–74 years who have missed work because of headache in previous year by pattern of headache (percentage in brackets)

Pattern	Total
Headache only	
Number in group	192
Number of men missing work	0 (0)
Number of days lost[1]	0
Headache + 1 feature	
Number in group	201
Number of men missing work	9 (4)
Number of days lost[1]	30
Headache + 2 features	
Number in group	175
Number of men missing work	14 (8)
Number of days lost[1]	57
Headache + 3 features	
Number in group	87
Number of men missing work	19 (22)
Number of days lost[1]	67
All headaches	
Number in group	655
Number of men missing work	42 (6)
Number of days lost[1]	154

[1] 16 of the 42 men missing work lost an unspecified number of additional days.

proportion seeking medical advice was also similar to that in previous surveys. In the Pontypridd area the proportion of those with headaches consulting a doctor in the previous year was 13% in men and 20% in women. In Southampton the corresponding figures were 12 and 19%.

Although the wording of many of the questions was identical to those of earlier studies [WATERS, 1974a, b] an attempt was made to improve some of them. Most importantly in earlier surveys the actual wording of the question about warning was identical to that in the present survey (fig. 1) but simply required a 'Yes' or 'No' answer. If 'Yes', the respondent was requested to describe briefly what was noticed. The replies were then examined individually and classified into various warning symptoms changes in mood, etc., minor visual aura, major visual aura, nausea, vomiting and paraesthesia). It was thought desirable to modify this in two ways for the Southampton study. Firstly, the respondent was asked if the

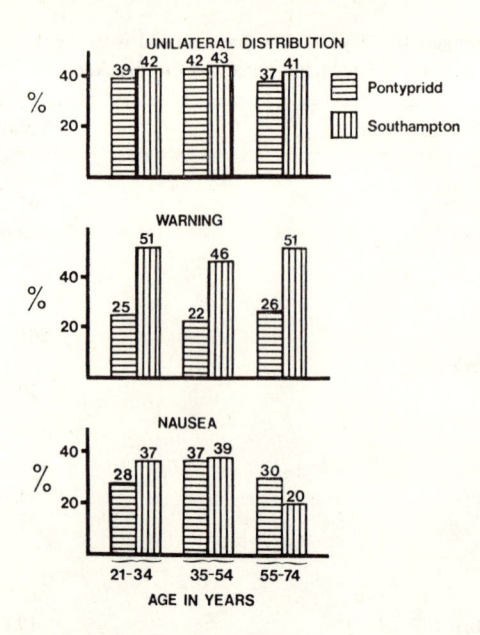

Fig. 7. Prevalence of three features of migraine in previous year in men with headache in Pontypridd and Southampton surveys. (Note: the context of the warning question was different in the two surveys.)

warning occurred 'sometimes', 'usually' or 'always' with headaches. This was to differentiate those with migraine attacks only and those who had other headaches between migraines. Similar wording about the frequency of the symptoms had been used in the past for other questions (e.g. unilateral distribution). Secondly, the various types of warning were listed (a to g in fig. 1) and the respondents chose the one(s) that applied. This could then be coded and analysed without being interpreted individually. It seemed that these were worthwhile improvements although it is well known that minor alterations in questions, even altering their order, can change the pattern of response. This is the most likely reason for the much higher prevalence of warning found in the Southampton survey. A comparison of the prevalence of the three features of migraine, amongst those with headache in the previous year, for the 1968 Pontypridd survey and the present Southampton survey is shown for men in figure 7 and for women in figure 8. The percentage with unilateral distribution and with nausea accompanying the headache is similar both in men and in women, in the two surveys. But warning is much more prevalent in the Southampton

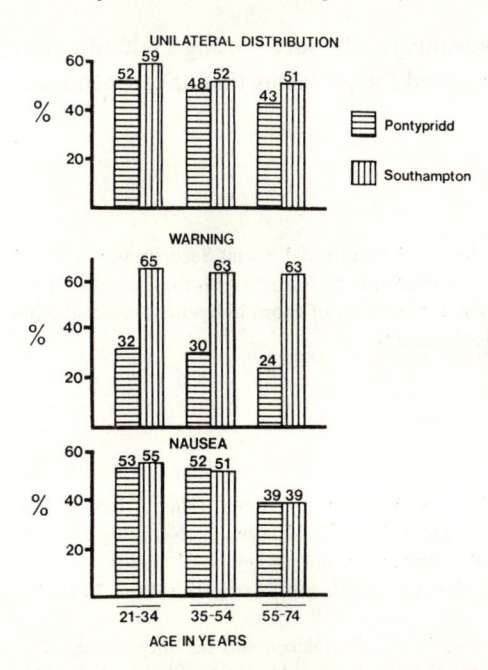

Fig. 8. Prevalence of three features of migraine in previous year in women with headache in Pontypridd and Southampton surveys (Note: the content of the warning question was different in the two surveys.)

survey. While it could be that warnings of headaches are more common in the city of Southampton this seems unlikely as the other features of migraine are equally prevalent. Earlier studies in widely differing populations showed a fairly uniform prevalence of headache and of the features of migraine once any differences in the age and sex composition of the populations was taken into account [WATERS, 1974a]. In view of this difference in the warning question, it is probably not appropriate to use the previous clinical validation of the original question [WATERS and O'CONNOR, 1970, 1971] to calculate the prevalence of migraine. However, as a continuing part of the present study two neurologists are attempting to diagnose migraine directly from the replies on the questionnaire and this diagnosis is then being validated in various sub-groups by the neurologists examining the subjects clinically. At present the results of the survey are presented without trying to establish the prevalence of migraine.

This survey has again shown the importance of headache in the general population. It has emphasised the fact that only a minority of sufferers consult their doctors and that the time off work due to this symptom is substantial. It has shown the advantages of a survey using a self-administered questionnaire and has demonstrated the problems that arise when trying to improve the questions.

Acknowledgements

We are grateful to the Department of Health and Social Security in London for a grant to finance this survey and to ALAN STANDFORD for help with the analysis. The survey could not have been undertaken without the help of those individuals selected from the community who completed the questionnaires.

References

BILLE, B.: Migraine in school children. Acta paediat. *51:* suppl. 136, pp. 1–51 (1962).
BREWIS, M.; POSKANZER, D.C.; ROLLAND, C., and MILLER, H.: Neurological disease in an English city. Acta neurol. scand. *42:* suppl. 24, pp. 1–84 (1966).
CHILDS, A.J. and SWEETNAM, M.T.: A study of 104 cases of migraine. Br. J. Ind. Med. *18:* 234–236 (1961).
DALSGAARD-NIELSON, T. and ULRICH, M.D.: Prevalence and heredity of migraine and migranoid headaches among 461 Danish doctors. Headache *12:* 168–172 (1973).
FITZ-HUGH, T.: Praecordial migraine: an important form of angina innocens. New int. Clin. *1:* 141–147 (1940).
Office of Health Economics: Migraine. Studies on current health problems (London 1972).
Office of Population, Censuses and Surveys: Enumeration district data (unpubl., 1966).
Office of Population, Censuses and Surveys: Classification of occupation (HMSO, 1970).
Office of Population, Censuses and Surveys: Registrar General's Revised Estimate of the Population for England and Wales in 1969 (HMSO, 1975).
SCOTT, C.: Research on mail surveys. J.R. Stat. Soc. *124:* 143–205 (1962).
WATERS, W.E.: Community studies of the prevalence of headache. Headache *9:* 178–186 (1970).
WATERS, W.E.: Migraine: intelligence, social class and familial prevalence. Br. med. J. *ii:*77–81 (1971).
WATERS, W.E. (ed.): The epidemiology of migraine (Boehringer, Ingelheim 1974a).
WATERS, W.E.: The Pontypridd Headache Survey. Headache *14:* 81–90 (1974b).
WATERS, W.E. and O'CONNOR, P.J.: Clinical validation of a headache questionnaire; in Background to migraine. 3rd Migraine Symposium, pp. 1–8 (Heinemann, London 1970).
WATERS, W.E. and O'CONNOR, P.J.: Epidemiology of headache and migraine in women. J. Neurol. Neurosurg. Psychiat. *34:* 148–153 (1971).
World Federation of Neurology's Research Group on Migraine and Headache: Editorial comment. Hemicrania *1:*3 (1969).

W.E. WATERS, Professor of Community Medicine, South Academic Block, Southampton General Hospital, *Southampton SO9 4XY* (England).

The Epidemiology and Genetics of Migraine

Dewey K. Ziegler

Department of Neurology, University of Kansas Medical Center,
College of Health Sciences and Hospital, Kansas City, Kans.

The definition of migraine is a controversial subject. It is best, therefore, temporarily to bypass this problem and review the data on the prevalence of headache as it has been studied in various populations.

It is a matter of common knowledge that headache is a common affliction. Ranking high as a cause for visits to physicians' offices [National Ambulatory Medical Care Survey, National Disease and Therapeutic Index, 1976], headache is the basis for a large market in over-the-counter pharmaceuticals. The exact numerical prevalence in the United States and the British Isles began to be studied in the 20th century. Weider et al. reported in 1944 that 87 of a group of 1,000 candidates presenting for induction into the armed services (presumably all males) gave a history of headache. More recent studies, with few exceptions, have reported much higher frequencies. (Perhaps the military doctors were not too eager to elicit this history.) Ogden [1952] studied 4,634 individuals comprising three groups: one of hospital employees, a second of highly educated individuals (medical and clergy), and a third group of individuals from various middle and lower socioeconomic backgrounds. Over all, 64.8% gave a history of having had headache (with no further details). Waters and his group have studied various epidemiologic aspects of headache and migraine during the past decade. Their instrument, a postal questionnaire, asked about events in the preceding year. In the original community survey of the population of a community [The Pontypridd Headache Survey, Waters, 1974b], they found extremely high percentages of individuals admitting to headache in this time period – up to 92% of women in the 21–34 age group and 74% of the men, with the percentages remaining higher for women and dropping as older age groups were sampled (fig. 1). These high figures have been

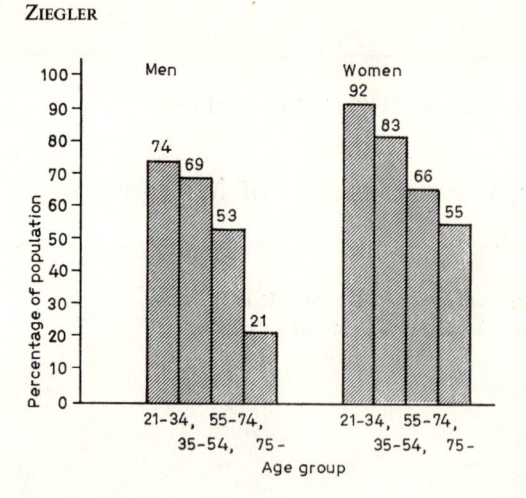

Fig. 1. Prevalence of headache in the year immediately before the 1968 Pontypridd survey. From WATERS [1975a].

found in several other groups studied by WATERS and co-workers, e.g., physicians in general practice [WATERS, 1975b] and groups from other geographical areas in the British Isles. Very similar figures have been reported from America. MARKUSH *et al.* [1975], using an interviewing technique, reported the occurrence of headache in 76.5% of their population of 451 women aged 25–44 (a control group for another study) for the previous year. ZIEGLER *et al.* [1977] obtained data from a self-administered questionnaire given to 1,809 volunteer non-clinic subjects varying in age from 16 to 70. This questionnaire asked whether the subject 'had ever been subject to headaches', thus involving an indefinite time period. Between 80 and 90% of the entire sample stated they had been subject to headaches, with figures for women and men being about equal. Approximately half of these subjects of both sexes, however, stated they had been subject only to mild headaches. Severe or disabling headaches were admitted to by 40.9% of the men and 50.2% of the women.

It has been assumed throughout recent centuries that there is a syndrome 'migraine' and that there is a group of patients afflicted with this syndrome. Certainly several rather dramatic events occur in some patients with headache. Severe vomiting is frequent, and before many attacks there are unusual visual hallucinations, described with great care and accuracy by a series of 19th and 20th century scientists who suffered them [Migraine in Astronomers and Natural Philosophers, JARCHO, 1968]. And yet, there is little agreement among experts as to the parameters of a migraine syndrome and what is essential to the diagnosis. Severe headache occurring intermittently would seem to be the one indispensable characteristic, and yet 'migraine without headache' has been described [WHITTY and OXON, 1967]. Over the years, however, various combinations of the following variables have been used to diagnose migraine: (1) severe, intermittent pain; (2) unilateral pain; (3) nausea and/or vomiting with attacks; (4) neurological phenomena preceding attacks, most commonly distortions of vision but including paresthesiae, hemiparesis, ophthalmoplegia, aphasia and confusion; (5) positive family history, itself defined in various ways; (6) response to ergotamine, and (7) tenderness of the scalp.

To cite only a few of the many studies in recent times, CHILDS and SWEETNAM [1961] used 1, 3 and 4, but noted that 'some otherwise typical cases occurred in which prodromal symptoms were absent and not in all cases did nausea and vomiting occur; these cases were included in the series'. WALKER [1959] required 1, 2, and one of 3, 4, or 5. WOLFF [1963] stressed 5, 6, and 7. OSTFELD [1962] felt the only reliable and objective criteria was 6, and LANCE and ANTHONY [1966] used 1, 2, and 3. Others have used as defining criteria duration of headache, duration of illness, cyclic vomiting in childhood.

The formulation of a headache classification by the Ad Hoc Committee on Classification of Headache of the National Institute of Neurological Diseases and Blindness [1968] was meant to provide uniformity of definition, but many ambiguities remain. Given these varying definitions, ZIEGLER et al. [1972] attempted to discover in a given series of patients with severe headaches and in whom a set number of variables were recorded, whether a statistical procedure – principal components factor analysis – would produce one 'factor' with the clinical characteristics of migraine and other factors suggestive of our accepted clinical entities. Three resultant factors shared the foregoing clinical features usually ascribed to migraine, suggesting three different groups of cases.

It is, therefore, not surprising that a more or less intuitive clinical judgment has been the major criterion for the diagnosis of migraine [WATERS and O'CONNOR, 1971] and that estimates of prevalence have been productive of such varying figures. The earlier studies reported much lower figures than later surveys. GRIMES [1931] reported 8% of a population of 15,000 with migraine, and WALKER [1959] in a careful study of 5,785 medical records and interviews with those suspected of migraine reported an incidence of 4.85%. CHILDS and SWEETNAM [1961] found 6.5% of 1,607 respondees to their questionnaire to have probable migraine, but the response rate was low. BREWIS *et al.* [1966], in a careful interview study of a sample population of an urban area, reported a 'migraine-like syndrome' (not further defined) in 3.3% and 'repeated headaches which have caused loss of time from work and school' in 6.2%. OGDEN [1952], using varying numbers of the criteria enumerated above, in his survey found 8.6% when 'migraine was broadly defined' – 3.3% when migraine was 'rigidly defined'.

Some more recent surveys, however, have reported migraine in much higher numbers. WATERS has studied large numbers of various population groups with a standardized questionnaire [WATERS and O'CONNOR, 1970]. Subsequently, samples of respondent populations who gave affirmative answers to questions covering headache and varying combinations of the following features – unilateral location, nausea and vomiting, warning – were interviewed. The percentage of respondents giving positive responses on the questionnaire on questions regarding 'migraine characteristics' to those adjudged by the physician on interview to have migraine was then calculated and the results extrapolated to the larger population groups. Using these techniques, he arrives at figures of prevalence rates for migraine of 23–24% in women and 15–20% in men. WATERS suggests that the lower values of earlier investigators may have been due to 'patients with migraine not attending their general practitioners, to the lack of a suitable definition of the condition, or to a poor response rate in the survey' [WATERS and O'CONNOR, 1971]. Yet, at least two surveys [OGDEN, 1952; BREWIS *et al.*, 1966] did not depend on patient response and criteria for migraine were not notably restrictive. MARKUSH, however, in a random sample of women, ages 15–44, also reported 23% having two or more symptoms of migraine headache during the year prior to interview. Finally, the survey of ZIEGLER *et al.* [1977] reports from a questionnaire study concerning life histories of a large non-clinic population the concurrence of 'migraine' phenomena with headache. 50% of the large population reporting disabling or severe headache, or about 20–25% of the whole population studied, had premonitory warning – a figure close to that of WATERS for migraine prevalence. Similar, but smaller, figures occurred for concurrence of unilateral character of headache and nausea occurring with disabling or severe headache. But of particular importance was the finding that 'migraine' phenomena occur with headaches rated as 'mild': warning phenomena in 22% of females, 20% of males; unilateral character in 12% of females, 11% of males.

What can be said, then, of the definition of the migraine syndrome? WATERS [1973] points to the increasing number of migraine symptoms reported with increase in severity of headache and suggests that in many patients the 'syndrome' is a nonspecific tendency to admit to symptoms, possibly correlated with neuroticism – a provocative idea. He admits, however, that apart from this nonspecific 'non-syndrome' there may well be a small 'true syndrome'. It is apparent, however, that important data are still lacking. We still do not know, for example, how consistently the features ordinarily considered diagnostic of migraine are associated. The study of ZIEGLER et al. [1972] has suggested that even when patients describe their headache attacks in the aggregate, there are confusing complexes of symptoms not consistent with our usual classification. More to the point, over a period of time, we do not know patterns of headache symptoms and their variability. Knowledge of such patterns is essential to evaluation of therapy. What, for example, is the incidence of prolonged remission in migraine? Does the patient have symptoms during this period and if so, what kind of symptoms?

Certain other epidemiological facts are more well established than that of the overall prevalence of migraine. All studies have shown that severe headaches are more frequent in the female than in the male [BREWIS et al., 1966; OGDEN, 1952; WALKER, 1959; WATERS, 1974]. Studies by BILLE [1962] in children have been of particular interest. In an excellent study of 9,059 school children and using carefully defined criteria, this author found the percentage of diagnosable migraine to rise from 1% in the age 6 group to 5% at age 15. No sex difference was apparent until age 11; above that age a highly significant preponderance in females appeared. It has been suggested in the past that the preponderance of migraine in females might be solely the result of more frequent utilization of medical facilities by women [OSTFELD, 1962], but the change in sex occurrence in early adolescence appears to negate this hypothesis. Studies of community samples have also confirmed the fact that severe headache is reported more often by women whether or not a physician is consulted [OGDEN, 1952; WATERS, 1974b; ZIEGLER et al., 1977].

The reason for the preponderance in women is obscure. The onset of the sex difference about the time of puberty suggests a relationship to hormones, and indeed 'menstrual migraine' has been described, and a relationship of migraine to the time of falling hormonal levels has been described [SOMERVILLE, 1972]. The latter is uncommon, however, and the preponderance of severe headache in women remains into postmenopausal years [WATERS, 1975a; ZIEGLER et al., 1977]. Again, the data suggest multiple factors favoring the concurrence of various kinds of headache in women.

That severe headache, or migraine by any definition, decreases with advancing age is attested to by most surveys, although one recent study found no decrease in women in any age group from 15 to 44 [MARKUSH et al., 1975]. This finding again raises the possibility of hormonal influences on the occurrence of migraine, and indeed many observers have recorded that migrainous women tend to show striking decreases in migraine with menopause, although one study does not confirm this [BREWIS et al., 1966].

Although the prevalence of severe headache drops with age, what appears to be a typical migrainous disturbance can appear in the fifth decade of life, and even later. How frequently this occurs is unknown, although WATERS [1975a] has shown that the prevalence of three features of migraine (unilaterality, nausea, warning) decline, in women, with age.

An intriguing question is whether the prevalence of migraine is the same worldwide. It appears that epidemiological studies on headache of any size have been carried out only in Britain, Scandinavia and the United States. The overall figures for all three areas are surprisingly similar, and recent figures for the occurrence of headache in non-clinic populations of WATERS and ZIEGLER are particularly close, although the actual wording of the survey questions was somewhat different. Whether the figures for the prevalence of headache differ, and if specific headache patterns occur in other cultures, particularly in the strikingly different ones of Africa and Asia, would be a subject of great interest and importance. In America, the only evidence for different ethnic groups has been provided by MARKUSH et al. [1975] who found somewhat higher figures for the prevalence of migraine among black women than among white.

It has long been thought that migraine is associated with high intelligence [AIRING, 1962; ALVAREZ, 1947; CALLAGHAN, 1968; SELINSKY, 1939; SIMPSON, 1968]. However, two recent studies have cast doubt on this association. WATERS [1971] studied the intelligence of four groups selected from a general population: one with migraine, a second with nonmigrainous headache, a third with unilateral headache, and a fourth with no headache. There was no significant difference in intelligence in the four groups. MARKUSH et al. [1975] studied headache in a random sample of 451 women and found that the less educated subjects reported significantly more migraine symptoms than the better educated.

It has also been generally thought that migraine is characteristic of upper socioeconomic classes, although CHILDS and SWEETNAM pointed out years ago that the disabling nature of migraine attacks would probably be more conspicuous in a 'managerial' group than in one of manual laborers. WATERS [1971] studied the social class of a random sample of 414 individuals and found no evidence for an increased amount of headache or migraine in the higher social classes, but rather an indication that the latter were more likely to consult a doctor for their symptoms.

The problem of the relationship of migraine to hypertension and vascular disease is difficult and controversial. The early studies of JANEWAY [1913] and of GARDNER et al. [1940] reported high percentages of the occurrence of migraine in hypertensive patients. WALKER, in his general practice population of 5,785 patients found a blood pressure that was 'higher than average for the population' among migraine patients, and particularly over the age of 50 there was a 'clear and possibly direct correlation between migraine and essential hypertension'.

OSTFELD [1962] and WOLFF [1963] could find no difference in the incidence and severity of headache in a hypertensive and control population, but they report a particular type of headache almost peculiar to the hypertensive population, and particularly to the patients with severe hypertension. LEVITON et al. [1974] found, in parents of migrainous patients, hypertension to be 1.7 times greater in a parent with migraine than one without. (They found also, incidentally, a greater risk of myocardial infarction in the migrainous parents.) MARKUSH et al. [1975] in their community study of young women found a highly significant association of hypertension with migraine, and ZIEGLER et al. [1977] also found a significant increase in reported hypertension by women with disabling or severe headache over those denying such headache.

Only two studies provide negative data on this subject. DOUGLAS [1964] concluded that there is no correlation between headache and hypertension unless the diastolic blood pressure is over 130 mm Hg, but his data show severe headache occurring in 15 of 89 patients with a diastolic pressure over 110 mm Hg. WATERS [1974a], in his community study, did not confirm a higher average systolic or diastolic blood pressure in any group admitting to headache or migraine than in those without such a history, but the number of his patients, particularly in the older age groups, was very small.

The problem of the genetics of migraine is clearly connected to that of the definition of the term. It is difficult to compare various studies done in the past, since varying criteria have been used; and the previous paragraphs have documented the extreme frequency of the headache symptom and the persistent difficulty of isolating 'migraine' from this population.

Observation of the frequent positive family history of headache dates as far back as LIVEING in the 19th century. All physicians who deal with headache patients have frequently encountered families in which several

Table I. Percent positive family history for headache

	Migraine	Control
Lennox	61.0 (parents only)	11.0 (parents only)
Sweetnam and Childs	36.5	5.8
Bille (children only)	72.6 (mothers)	17.8 (parents or siblings)
	20.5 (fathers)	
		($p<0.01$)

generations have suffered from headache with features of migraine [Allen, 1930; Barolin, 1970; Barolin and Sperlich, 1969; Refsum, 1968]. Because of these pedigrees, the mechanism of inheritance has been assumed by some to be dominant [Allen, 1930; Christiansen, 1925]. Goodell and Wolff, however, felt that the data were more consistent with a hypothesis of recessivity. Dalsgaard-Nielsen [1965], in another review of the literature and from personal experience, considers it probable that the 'basis for heredity is complicated, possibly with an additive effect of numerous genes, similar to the state of affairs regarding the rule of inheritance of epilepsy'. Barolin [1970] also entertains the possibility of 'multiple allelism being active in determining the inheritance of migraine', and also presents data suggesting a dominant mode of inheritance with greater penetration in females, the genes being expressed either by migraine or cerebral dysrhythmia. These reports indicate the complexity of the genetic problem.

Three controlled studies have provided figures of the familial incidence of headache in migraine patients, considerably in excess of those without headache. These results are tabulated in table I.

A dissenting report is that of Waters [1971] who administered a questionnaire to 524 immediate relatives of a small random sample (155 individuals) of a community; these individuals had been identified from a previous study as having no headache history, nonmigrainous or migraine. The prevalence of migraine in the families of migraine patients was 10%, and 5–6% in the other groups – a difference that was not statistically significant. Waters points out that other studies have contained possible biases, in particular the one of accepting a case as migraine *if* there is a positive family history.

Comparison of monozygotic and dizygotic twins is one of the standard methods of searching for a possible genetic trait. Twin studies of this subject have been few, and the important and often difficult problem of determining zygosity has often not been possible to solve. The twin material of EBBING [1956] consisted of an unselected series of pairs. Although 3 were diagnosed as monozygotic pairs and 10 dizygotic, the methods of determining zygosity were ill-defined. One of the three monozygotic pairs was concordant for typical migraine and 3 of 10 dizygotic, an almost identical percentage in this small group. Other nontypical migraine headache occurred in the other two monozygotic pairs, and in three additional dizygotic pairs. HARVALD and HAUGE [1956] reviewed records of an unselected series of 1,900 pairs of twins. It is stated that 'attempts were made to confirm the zygosity diagnosis by examination of blood groups', or by review of old photographs and information from relatives. Subjects were asked whether there had been admission to the hospital for severe illness, including migraine. Concordance was found in 6 of 18 probably monozygotic pairs, and 3 of 54 probably dizygotic pairs. It should be borne in mind that these were hospitalized individuals and that criteria for zygosity were again variable. In this study whose numbers are clearly indicative of a preponderance of concordance in monozygotic pairs, no clinical details are given to support the diagnosis of migraine. More recently, PEMBREY [1972] has recorded a carefully studied monozygotic twin pair discordant for migraine.

Most recently, ZIEGLER *et al.* [1975] interviewed 106 unselected twin pairs in all of whom zygosity was carefully documented by extensive blood grouping, and by evaluation of height, weight, appearance and answers to a series of questions concerning judgment as to similarity. 65 twin pairs were judged to be dizygotic, and 41 monozygotic. The subjects were interviewed and data gathered as to whether they had been subject to severe or disabling headache (criteria were supplied). Other data on specific clinical phenomena relevant to the diagnosis of migraine were also gathered, but it was assumed that if an individual denied having been subject to severe headache, he or she had *not* had migraine; and that conversely, all migraine patients (plus, possibly, some others as per the difficulties of diagnosis) would fall in the group admitting to disabling or severe headache. Of the 82 individuals comprising 41 monozygotic twin pairs, there were 11 giving a history of severe or disabling headache, two sets of concordant twins and seven individuals discordant for the symptom. The overall frequency of concordance was almost identical in monozygotic and in dizygotic, same-sex twin pairs (2 concordant pairs, 8 discordant). This result clearly casts doubt on a genetic component in headache occurring in, at least, a large number of these pairs.

REFSUM, after reviewing all available twin data up to 1968 concluded, 'the results of these studies seem to indicate clearly that genetic factors are not the sole determinant for the manifestation of migraine'. These words are clearly true and probably a considerable understatement.

Two points must be made concerning genetics of migraine. As several authors have pointed out in the past, the problem of differentiating patterns of behavior and symptomatology 'learned' in early childhood from true genetic influence is a formidable one. Sorting out these influences is best done by studying groups of symptomatic individuals who have, and groups who have not, been raised by the natural parents, as has been done by KETY et al. [1968] for schizophrenia. No similar study, of course, has been undertaken in migraine.

Secondly, whatever may be inherited is clearly not a headache, but rather a type of physiological or psychological reaction to various environmental influences. Again, several authors have pointed to this fact in the past, but the extreme difficulties of searching for these possible objective traits in families have understandably not been surmounted. There are possibly several complex sets of facts consisting of genetic predispositions and appropriate 'releasing' environmental stimuli – the mechanism documented so extensively in lower animals in recent years [TINBERGEN, 1969]. There are at least many clues as to identifiable disordered functions in patients with migraine. They include 'vasomotor instability' [APPENZELLER et al., 1963], reaction of the central nervous system to photic stimuli [RICHEY et al., 1966] and abnormal behavior of blood platelets [SJAASTAD, 1975], to mention a few. In the presence of the inherited predisposition, certain individuals may have headache precipitated by various types of stress, fasting [BLAU and CUMINGS, 1966], ingestion of certain food substances [SANDLER et al., 1970], or variation in hormonal levels [SOMERVILLE, 1972]. Study of one or more of these functions in patients and their immediate relatives, in parallel with study of the headache symptom, should provide fertile fields for research.

References

Ad Hoc Committee on Classification of Headache of the National Institute of Neurological Diseases and Blindness: Classification of headache; in VINKEN and BRUYN Handbook of clinical neurology, vol. 5, pp. 11–14 (North-Holland, Amsterdam 1968).

AIRING, C.D.: Vascular headache. The headache associated with 'vasomotor instability'. Am. Heart J. 64: 715–716 (1962).

ALLEN, W.: The inheritance of migraine. Archs. intern. Med. *13:* 590–599 (1930).
ALVAREZ, W.C.: The migrainous personality and constitution. The essential features of the disease. A study of 500 cases. Am. J. med. Sci. *213:* 1–7 (1947).
APPENZELLER, O.; DAVISON, K., and MARSHALL, J.: Reflex vasomotor abnormalities in the hands of migrainous subjects. J. Neurol. Neurosurg. Psychiat. *26:* 447–450 (1963).
BAROLIN, G.S.: in COCHRANE Background to migraine. 3rd Migraine Symposium, pp. 28–37 (Heinemann, London 1970).
BAROLIN, G.S. und SPERLICH, D.: Migränefamilien. Fortschr. Neurol. Psychiat. *37:* 521–544 (1969).
BILLE, B.: Migraine in school children. Acta pediat. *51:* suppl. 136, pp. 1–151 (1962).
BLAU, J.N. and CUMINGS, J.N.: Method of precipitating and preventing some migraine attacks. Br. med. J. *ii:* 1242–1243 (1966).
BREWIS, M.; POSKANZER, D.C.; ROLLAND, C., et al.: Neurological disease in an English city. Acta neurol. scand. *42:* suppl. 24, pp. 1–89 (1966).
CALLAGHAN, N.: The migraine syndrome in pregnancy. Neurology *18:* 197–199 (1968).
CHILDS, A.J. and SWEETNAM, M.T.: A study of 104 cases of migraine. Br. J. Indust. Med. *18:* 234–236 (1961).
CHRISTIANSEN, V.: Rapport sur la migraine. Revue neurol. *32:* 855–881 (1925).
DALSGAARD-NIELSEN, T.: Migraine and heredity. Acta neurol. scand. *41:* 287–300 (1965).
DELOZIER, J.E.: National Ambulatory Medical Care Survey. DHEW Publication No. (HRA) 76–1772 (1976).
DOUGLAS, R.M.: Hypertension and headache. A survey of 231 treated hypertensive patients. N.Z. med. J. *63:* 70–76 (1964).
EBBING, H.C.: Migräne bei Zwillingen, vorläufige Mitteilung. Acta Genet. med. Gemell. *5:* 371–382 (1956).
GARDNER, J.W.; MOUNTAIN, G.E., and HINES, E.A.: The relationship of migraine to hypertension and hypertension headaches. Am. J. med. Sci. *200:* 50–53 (1940)
GOODELL, H.; LEWONTIN, R., and WOLFF, H.G.: Familial occurrence of migraine headache. A study of heredity. Archs. Neurol. Psychiat. *72:* 325–334 (1954).
GRIMES, E.: The migraine instability. Med. J. Rec. *134:* 417–422 (1931).
HARVALD, B. and HAUGE, M.: A catamnestic investigation of Danish twins. A preliminary report. Dan. med. Bull. *3:* 150–158 (1956).
JANEWAY, T.C.: A clinical study of hypertensive cardiovascular disease. Archs intern. Med. *12:* 755–798 (1913).
JARCHO, S.: Migraine in astronomers and 'natural philosophers'. Bull. N.Y. Acad. Med. *44:* 886–891 (1968).
KETY, S.S.; ROSENTHAL, D.; WENDER, P.H., and SCHULSINGER, F.: The types of prevalence of mental illness in the biological and adoptive families of adopted schizophrenics; in KETY and ROSENTHAL Transmission of schizophrenia (Pergamon Press, Oxford 1968).
LANCE, J.W. and ANTHONY, M.: Some clinical aspects of migraine. A prospective survey of 500 patients. Archs Neurol. *15:* 356–361 (1966).
LEVITON, A.; MALVEA, B., and GRAHAM, J.R.: Vascular diseases, mortality, and migraine in the parents of migraine patients. Neurology *24:* 669–672 (1974).
LIVEING, E.: On megrim, sick-headache and some allied disorders (Churchill, London 1873).

Markush, R.E.; Karp, H.R.; Heyman, A., and O'Fallon, W.M.: Epidemiologic study of migraine symptoms in young women. Neurology 25: 430–435 (1975).

National Disease and Therapeutic Index, Report of 1976 (Lea Associates, Amoler).

Ogden, H.D.: Headache studies: statistical data. Procedure and sample distribution. J. Allergy 23: 58–75 (1952).

Ostfeld, A.M.: The common headache syndromes (Thomas, Springfield 1962).

Pembrey, M.E.: Discordant identical twins. Practitioner 209: 846 (1972).

Refsum, S.: Genetic aspects of migraine; in Vinken and Bruyn Handbook of clinical neurology, vol. 5, pp. 258–269 (North-Holland, Amsterdam 1968).

Richey, E.T.; Kooi, K.A., and Waggoner, R.W.: Visually evoked responses in migraine. Electroenceph. clin. Neurophysiol. 21: 23–27 (1966).

Sandler, M.; Youdim, M.B.H.; Southgate, J., and Hanington, E.: in Cochrane Background to migraine. 3rd Migraine Symposium, pp. 103–112 (Heinemann, London 1970).

Selinsky, H.: Psychological study of the migrainous syndrome. Bull. N.Y. Acad, Med. 15: 757–763 (1939).

Simpson, J.A.: in Dunlop Textbook of medical treatment (Livingstone, Edinburgh 1968).

Sjaastad, O.: The Significance of blood serotonin levels in migraine. Acta neurol. scand. 51: 200–210 (1975).

Somerville, B.W.: The influence of hormones upon migraine in women. Med. J. Aust., ii: special suppl., pp. 6–11 (1972).

Tinbergen, N.: The study of instinct (Oxford University Press, Oxford 1969).

Walker, C.H.: Migraine and its relationship to hypertension. Br. med. J. ii: 1430–1433 (1959).

Waters, W.E.: Migraine: intelligence, social class, and familial prevalence. Br. med. J. ii: 77–81 (1971).

Waters, W.E.: The epidemiological enigma of migraine. Int. J. Epidem. 2: 189–194 (1973).

Waters, W.E.: The epidemiology of migraine (Boehringer Ingelheim, Bracknell 1974a).

Waters, W.E.: The Pontypridd Headache Survey. Headache 14: 81–90 (1974b).

Waters, W.E.: Epidemiological data relevant to prognosis in migraine in adults. Int. J. Epidem. (1975a).

Waters, W.E.: Migraine in general practitioners. Br. J. prev. Soc. Med. 29: 48–52 (1975b).

Waters, W.E. and O'Connor, P.J.: Clinical validation of a headache questionnaire; in Cochrane Background to migraine. 3rd Migraine Symposium, pp. 1–8 (Heinemann, London 1970).

Waters, W.E. and O'Connor, P.J.: Epidemiology of headache and migraine in women. J. Neurol. Neurosurg. Psychiat. 34: 148–153 (1971).

Weider, A.; Mittlemann, B.; Wechsler, D., and Wolff, H.G.: The Cornell Selectee Index. A method for quick testing of selectees for the armed forces. J. Am. med. Ass. 124: 224–228 (1944).

Whitty, C.W.M. and Oxon, D.M.: Migraine without headache. Lancet ii: 283–285 (1967).

Wolff, H.G.: Headache and other head pain; 2nd ed. (Oxford University Press, New York 1963).

ZIEGLER, D.K.; HASSANEIN, R., and HASSANEIN, K.: Headache syndromes suggested by factor analysis of symptom variables in a headache prone population. J. chron. Dis. 25: 353–363 (1972).
ZIEGLER, D.K.; HASSANEIN, R.S.; HARRIS, D., and STEWART, R.: Headache in a nonclinic twin population. Headache 14: 213–218 (1975).
ZIEGLER, D.K.; HASSANEIN, R.S., and COUCH, J.R.: Characteristics of life headache histories in a nonclinic population. Neurology 27: 265–269 (1977).

DEWEY K. ZIEGLER, MD, Professor and Chairman, Department of Neurology, University of Kansas Medical Center, 3900 Rainbow Boulevard, *Kansas City, KS 66103* (USA)

Migraine in Childhood

CHARLES F. BARLOW

Children's Hospital Medical Center, Department of Neurology, Harvard Medical School, Boston, Mass.

Contents

Introduction	34
Substrate of Childhood Migraine	36
Expression of Childhood Migraine	37
Common Migraine	37
Classic Migraine	37
Cyclic Vomiting	37
Abdominal Migraine	38
Convulsions Associated with Migraine	38
Ophthalmoplegic Migraine	38
Hemiplegic Migraine, including Aphasia and Focal Somatic Sensory Phenomena	39
Basilar Artery Migraine	39
Confusional States	40
Benign Paroxysmal Vertigo	40
Paroxysmal Leg Pain	41
Psychogenic Headaches	41
Symptomatic Vascular Headaches – Differential Diagnosis and Ancillary Studies	41
Treatment	43
Prognosis	44
References	45

Introduction

The various manifestations of migraine are a common problem of childhood, with estimates that approximately 4% of unselected school children between age 7 and 15 are affected [BILLE, 1962.] There is a lesser incidence in earlier years. Although probably accurate, this incidence is greater than most practicing pediatricians would estimate. The full range of the subject is not extensively discussed in most pediatric textbooks, nor is there an extensive literature. It would be agreed that headaches, and to a lesser extent, periodic vomiting are common enough, but a psychogenic etiology is given first priority, not migraine. In fact, psychogenic headaches are rare before adolescence, and vascular headaches are far more common. It follows that there is a tendency to underdiagnose migraine phenomena in childhood. Emphasis on the emotional aspect is not entirely out of place, however, inasmuch as it is the most common factor which aggravates both the frequency and severity of the problem.

The essential clinical characteristics of juvenile migraine are similar to migrainic symptoms in adult life. Symptoms may begin at any age, and the onset of puzzling episodic symptoms at age 2–3 years is reasonably common in retrospective histories. Onset is usually later in childhood, however. The chief feature is periodicity of recurrence, that is, an on and off quality. Frequency varies from several times per week to several times per year. The duration of each paroxysmal episode is generally shorter than in adults, and is measured in portions of an hour to several hours as a rule, while more severe episodes of nausea and vomiting may last 1–2 days. This is in sharp contrast with the other common paroxysmal phenomena of childhood, seizures, which are usually measured in minutes. The predominant symptom is usually headache which has a throbbing quality and may be hemicranial, but is usually bitemporal-frontal. The vocabulary of early childhood does not allow for easy ascertainment of the history of throbbing quality, but it usually can be developed. Gesture language is sometimes helpful. Episodes can often be terminated by sleep or rest. The child usually becomes noticeably less active during an episode and often spontaneously seeks the quiet of couch or bedroom. Associated symptomatology which is most frequently present consists of anorexia, nausea, much less commonly vomiting, sometimes accompanied by abdominal pain. Either of the latter may dominate the clinical presentation leading to the designation 'cyclic vomiting' and 'abdominal migraine'. It is often possible for the parents to recognize when the child is having an attack by the appearance of facial pallor, rarely flushing, or by behavioral change which may be irritability or lethargy, and withdrawal. There may be evidence of photophobia, but other visual symptoms such as scotomata are not especially common. Children seem to be more prone than adults to complex neurologic phenomena, such as hemiparesis, aphasia, confusional states, vertigo, opthalmoplegia, and overt brain stem signs and symptoms.

Substrate of Childhood Migraine

The most significant background factor in childhood migraine is a family history, often enough on both the paternal and maternal sides. Incidence varies as given in the literature, but HOLGUIN and FENICHEL [1967] report 87%. It is probably 95% or more if the family history is carefully explored, and includes aunts, uncles, and grandparents. It is not sufficient to inquire of a history of 'migraine' or 'sick' headaches, because a different interpretation is often given and reference to 'sinus' or 'tension' headaches is frequent when the true basis is common migraine. The best approach is to take a headache history from the parents themselves, and begin with the statement, 'Now, tell me about *your* headaches'. Then proceed with a systematic inquiry regarding periodicity, throbbing quality, and associated symptoms such as anorexia or nausea in available parents and include a discussion of the headaches of other members of the family. It is well to be cautious when a family history cannot be developed in the patient who would seem to have migraine.

History of early and current motion sickness is also frequent in children with migraine [BILLE, 1962]. The incidence of this associated symptom is not known.

Psychogenic factors play a role in aggravating the frequency and severity of migraine in childhood. This association should not be confused with the basic cause, which would seem to be an inherited pathophysiologic vascular responsivity, the basis of which is not known. Assessment of environmental factors may be productive, and familial tensions and excessive extracurricular activities leading to anxiety or depressive reactions are reasonably frequent [LING, *et al.*, 1970]. Problems in school also turn up, and unrecognized specific learning disabilities appear to be a basis for emotional distress in a surprising number of children, especially boys. Attention to these factors can be valuable in management.

A discrete triggering event for an episode is rare, although 'allergy' as the basis of migraine appeals to some. When intake of certain foods, such as chocolate or glutamate in Chinese food, leads to migrainic symptoms, a better interpretation may be the presence of a biochemical provocateur rather than a hyperergic immune reaction. Some patients seem to respond to a postprandial or fasting trigger to their headache at times when relative hypoglycemia may be suspected. This is often associated with a mild confusional state which may be the predominating symptom.

Head trauma does seem to be an effective stimulus to migraine in some patients. This is best expressed in certain dramatic syndromes where transient blindness, hemiparesis, brain stem signs as well as headache, somnolence and vomiting develop after a short latent period of minutes to hours. A fairly extensive and convincing recent literature has developed on this topic [GREENBLATT, 1973; HAAS and SOVNER, 1969; HAAS et al., 1975].

Expression of Childhood Migraine

Common Migraine
The usual expression of migraine in childhood is periodic throbbing headache associated with some anorexia and nausea, as described somewhat more extensively in the introduction. All other forms are relatively less common.

Classic Migraine
Periodic hemicranial throbbing headaches associated with nausea and vomiting, preceded by visual scotomata, constitute the classic symptomatology of migraine. Even in adults it constitutes only 5–10% of vascular headaches. It appears with almost equal frequency in adolescence, but it less common in younger children.

Cyclic Vomiting
Among a number of specific disorders of the gastrointestinal system and nervous system (including emotional illness), the pediatric literature has recognized the syndrome of cyclic vomiting. This consists of recurrent episodes of nausea and vomiting, sometimes associated with abdominal pain and fever. The usual duration of the upset is hours, and less commonly, several days. As the duration lengthens, signs and symptoms of dehydration develop. Between attacks, the children are entirely normal, although they may also suffer from periodic headaches. The common age range is from 6 to 11 years, and frequency has been reported as 2–3% [CULLEN and MACDONALD, 1963]. Follow up studies have indicated that as many as 75% of children with cyclic vomiting develop migraine headaches in later childhood and early adult life [HAMMOND, 1974]. It is likely that childhood migraine is the basis of the majority of cases with the syndrome of cyclic vomiting.

Abdominal Migraine

This syndrome overlaps with that of cyclic vomiting, but is distinguished by the predominance of abdominal pain and the tendency to briefer episodes which are usually 5–10 min in duration and occasionally somewhat longer. The frequency has been reported at 5–6% of children [CULLEN and MACDONALD, 1963]. The syndrome has been the focal point of a recurring controversy in the literature in relation to abdominal epilepsy. Both phenomena exist, but migraine is much more common. Most convincing of abdominal epilepsy are those patients in whom the onset of symptoms is sudden, where the level of consciousness or mental status is altered, and the episode is no more than 2–3 min in duration. The diagnosis of abdominal epilepsy is supported by interictal paroxysmal epileptiform electroencephalographic discharges with sharp transients. The frequency of various electroencephalographic abnormalities in juvenile migraine may be a confounding factor in the diagnosis, and it is unwise to place undue emphasis on the electroencephalogram in making the distinction.

Convulsions Associated with Migraine

The concurrence of migraine and convulsive disorder in the same patient seems to happen with greater than chance frequency. It is perhaps not surprising that an inherited tendency to unduly excitable or poorly inhibited tissue involves both the nerve cells and blood vessels in some people. Of additional interest is the rare occurrence of convulsion during a fully developed migraine episode. It would seem that the vascular reaction triggers the convulsion in these instances. This sequence is part of the experience of a number of neurologists, but there is no very definitive literature on the subject. A seizure during migraine must be distinguished from syncope – a phenomenon which is reasonably frequent in migrainic patients, especially in adolescence.

Ophthalmoplegic Migraine

Episodic ophthalmoplegia usually involving the third nerve, much less commonly the sixth nerve, is a rare expression of migraine [FRIEDMAN, et al., 1962]. Early childhood onset is typical and the usual patient is age 2–4 at the time of the first attack. It is unusual for the first episode to occur in adult life. Ophthalmoplegia may or may not be associated with headache and nausea. There is great variation in the duration of ophthalmoplegia, which may last from days to weeks. Occasionally recovery is incomplete, especially after several episodes of ophthalmoplegia. Also variable is the frequency and periodicity of recurrence, as well as associated periodic vascular headache without ophthalmoplegia. The diagnosis is tenable only after angiographic and other studies reveal no alternative reason for headache and ophthalmoplegia, aneurysm in particular.

Hemiplegic Migraine, including Aphasia and
Focal Somatic Sensory Phenomena

Numbness about the mouth and in both hands, sometimes on only one side, is relatively common in adolescent and adult migraine, but one seldom hears of it from preadolescent patients. Hemiplegic weakness is even less frequent, and when on the appropriate side, may be accompanied by aphasia. The more common form develops during the prodrome of the headache and lasts several minutes. A second variety is more persistent and the onset is usually delayed until the headache is well established [ISLER, 1971]. The headache is usually severe in hemiplegic migraine, but may be quite mild and even overlooked or absent. Focal signs may persist for up to 10 days and still be reversible, but the usual duration is less than 24 h. Cerebrospinal fluid protein may be transiently elevated in these patients. Infarction with enduring signs is a rare complication [CONNOR, 1962]. In a series of 18 cases with permanent sequelae, CONNOR found hemispheric symptoms, particularly occipital, to be most common. There was considerably lesser incidence of retinal infarction, while brain stem infarction was least common. Of the 18 patients, 6 were 10–16 years of age at the time of the incident. VERRET and STEELE, [1971] have reported an incidence of 50% residual signs in a group of 8 patients whose hemiplegic migraine developed in infancy. Angiography during episodes may reveal no alteration of arterial caliber, spasm or dilatation [ISLER, 1971]. A particularly interesting issue in the group of hemiplegic migraines is the familial clustering of patients, and families have been encountered in whom the recurring hemiplegia is on the same side.

Basilar Artery Migraine

Just as the internal carotid circulation may express focal neurologic signs, so may the vertebral-basilar system [BICKERSTAFF, 1961]. In the classic instance, a medley of brain stem signs develops and the predominant symptoms may include dysarthria, ataxia, complex ophthalmoplegia, and facial weakness. Onset is often between 5 and 10 years, and episodes may continue into adult life. Familial basilar migraine may occur, and it seems to be more frequent in girls [GOLDEN and FRENCH, 1975]. The usual duration of an attack is up to 30 min, and deficits lasting days are most unusual.

Of course, hemianopsic phenomena of the prodrome of classic migraine relate to the territory of the posterior cerebral arteries which are the terminals of the basilar system. Occasional instances of transient or persisting hemianopsia occur more frequently than dysfunction lower in the system. Vertigo is an even more common accompaniment of migraine, so it is fair to say that fragments of vertebral-basilar dysfunction may be more common, although the fully developed syndrome of basilar migraine is rare.

Confusional States

Impairment of the sensorium leading to an acute confusional state has been reported in juveniles as an expression of migraine [GASCON and BARLOW, 1970]. Restless agitation, drowsiness, and some dysarthria may progress to stupor. The usual duration is from 2 to 12 h. On occasion, elements of aphasia are part of the clinical picture. Headache and nausea may be absent, or only recalled after the episode has subsided. The usual age range is mid-childhood through early adolescence, and boys seem to be more prone than girls. As in most of the complex migraine syndromes, periodic recurrences are infrequent. At onset, this diffuse cerebral syndrome must be distinguished from exogenous intoxication and endogenous metabolic disturbance, including hypoglycemia as well as minor status epilepticus, and viral encephalitis or other infectious processes. Elements of disordered mental status are common in migrainic phenomena at any age, but are usually a minor part of the clinical expression, while in these patients confusion and disorientation predominate.

Benign Paroxysmal Vertigo

The syndrome of 'benign paroxysmal vertigo' was defined by BASSER in 1964. It consists of brief, 1- to 4-min attacks of vertigo (often nystagmus is visible to parents) and ataxia in young children (usual onset 2–3 years), without alteration of consciousness. Neurologic examination is normal as is the electroencephalogram, although there is usually an abnormal vestibular caloric response. Hearing is normal and there is no tinnitus. Some children develop torticollis during the attack which may persist for hours [DUNN and SNYDER, 1976]. As indicated in the discussion of basilar migraine, vertigo is commonly experienced in the various migraine syndromes of childhood [WATSON and STEELE, 1974]. It usually is a brief incident in the longer paroxysm of vasomotor instability symptomatology, such as headache.

An early report [FENICHEL, 1967] suggested a high incidence of subsequent migraine in children with 'benign paroxysmal vertigo', a suggestion which has not been confirmed by follow up of larger series [DUNN and SNYDER, 1976; KOENIGSBERGER et al., 1970]. The characteristic caloric partial unresponsiveness may be the key feature which distinguishes the majority of children with true benign paroxysmal vertigo of unknown etiology, from the group where vertigo without headache is an expression of migraine.

Paroxysmal Leg Pain

Some migrainic children suffer from paroxysmal leg pain involving one or both legs. Episodes last from several minutes to an hour, and are not accompanied by palpable cramping as a rule. It probably represents a migraine equivalent, although the literature on the subject is not extensive [CULLEN and MACDONALD, 1963].

Psychogenic Headaches

Children prior to puberty may complain of abdominal pain or vomiting as a consequence of psychologic distress, but it is uncommon for them to emphasize headache. When psychogenic headaches occur, they have many of the features of the tension and psychogenic headaches of adolescents and adults. The headaches tend to be expressed as continual discomfort although it may wax and wane. The quality of the sensation is described as a constricting or pressing sensation located at the vertex or posteriorly. Of greatest importance are the associated symptoms of anxiety or depression, usually expressed by ancillary behavioral symptomatology or an overt depression of mood.

Symptomatic Vascular Headaches –
Differential Diagnosis and Ancillary Studies

All childhood migraine syndromes, including common periodic headache, may be symptomatic of structural abnormality of blood vessels or of intracranial tumor. The incidence of organic abnormality is very low, and the likelihood varies with the clinical expression, being higher when there are focal signs such as ophthalmoplegia, hemiplegia, aphasia, or brain stem dysfunction. Each clinical syndrome has a somewhat different differential diagnosis, with intracranial abnormalities predominating in the headache syndromes as well as in those with focal neurological signs. When periodic vomiting and abdominal pain dominate the clinical picture, one must also consider intra-abdominal disorders and even lead colic. Upper and lower gastrointestinal X-rays and examination and culture of stools are appropriate. The female heterozygote of the X-linked recessive ornithine transcarbamylase deficiency is subject to periodic headache, confusion and vomiting [BRUTON et al., 1970]. Elevated ammonia values during the attack, as well as brothers who become grossly handicapped in infancy, provide the clues. Pheochromocytoma with intermittent hypertensive crises should also be considered. When periodic ataxia is the major symptom, pyruvate decarboxylase deficiency could be the answer [BLASS, et al., 1970]. Porphyria may also cause episodic abdominal pain, sometimes associated with changes in mental status, but symptomatic porphyria is essentially unknown before puberty.

A careful examination is probably the best screening device, and considerable clinical reassurance is gained by a history of alternation of hemicrania or lateralized neurologic phenomena. The incidence of organic processes is well under 0.5% in any case, and inasmuch as one cannot perform arteriograms in every patient, some vascular anomalies will inevitably be missed. Ocular refractive errors may contribute to the frequency of migraine, but are not causal. Chronic sinusitis in childhood does not produce migraine or headache without direct evidence of sinus infection such as frontal or maxillary tenderness and postnasal discharge.

Regular skull X-rays are appropriate in all patients with childhood migraine, although the yield of abnormality is low. An electroencephalogram probably is not indicated in common migraine in childhood, although it is frequently abnormal in migrainic children, especially during an attack. The changes in asymptomatic periods consist primarily of theta slowing, sometimes with paroxysmal quality, most often observed in posterior leads. Complex hemispheric symptoms such as hemiplegia, hemianopsia and aphasia are usually associated with prominent focal slowing while diffuse slow waves of delta frequency are usual when confusion is the predominant symptom. These electroencephalographic changes during episodes are only an indication of distressed tissue, and are not diagnostic. A case has been made for a strong association with 14 and 6/second positive spikes and juvenile migraine [WHITEHOUSE et al., 1967]. This position is considerably weakened by the indication that this electroencephalographic configuration is an almost universal phenomenon of preadolescent and adolescent years [SCHWARTZ and LOMBROSO, 1968], an age which happens to coincide with increasing migraine frequency. True epileptic spike discharges can give differential weight to the concept of abdominal epilepsy if the clinical description is appropriate. When one discovers a persistent interparoxysmal focal slow focus, further neurodiagnostic studies are indicated.

Computerized tomography has provided a noninvasive method for intracranial study of patients with juvenile migraine. Experience is rapidly expanding, but we are as yet uncertain of its limitations, especially with regard to small parenchymal vascular malformations. The procedure can demonstrate only a few of the very largest congenital berry aneurysms. Certainly, it should be employed in all instances of complicated migraine, and in all instances where migraine and a convulsive disorder occur in the same patient, especially if the seizures have a focal clinical or electrical quality.

The addition of cerebral arteriography to computerized tomography scanning should settle almost all questions of structural anomalies, including aneurysm. Aneurysm is very rare in childhood, particularly as compared with the more common arteriovenous malformations and those occasional patients with occlusive vascular disease and episodic hemiplegic symptoms related to 'Moya-moya' revascularization. The syndromes of ophthalmoplegic migraine in particular and most instances of basilar artery migraine require arteriographic study. There is no definitive literature on the possible increased risk of arteriography in migrainic children, although there is concern that there may be increased risk of infarction, particularly in the acute phase. It is advisable to defer this study to an interictal period if possible.

Lumbar puncture is occasionally necessary in the acute phase of complicated episodes, especially in the confusional states, because of the possibility of encephalitis or early purulent meningitis. Cerebrospinal fluid protein may be transiently elevated in children with complicated migraine.

Treatment

Aspirin and other analgesics such as aspirin-butalbital combinations (Fiorinal) can be helpful in mild and moderately severe headaches. If the headache is infrequent, this may be all that is needed once the reassurance of a specific diagnosis is given. If a prodrome or buildup of headache of sufficient duration is common, then Cafergot (1 tablet every 30 min X3) or sublingual ergot preparations may be useful. There are great limitations in childhood, however, because younger children should not, and adolescents usually will not carry their medication with them at all times.

If headaches are sufficiently frequent and severe (weekly with some disruption of activity), or if the episodes are complex even if not particularly frequent, a trial period of prophylactic daily medication is in order. First choice favorites vary but include phenobarbital (30 mg b.i.d. or t.i.d.), phenytoin (50 mg b.i.d. or t.i.d.), and some prefer various antihistaminic preparations. Second order drugs include propranolol (10 mg t.i.d. or q.i.d.) [WEBER and REINMUTH, 1972] and amitriptyline (25 mg daily to 25 mg b.i.d.), [COUCH et al., 1976], which may be preferred if a depressive mood predominates. Imipramine may also be used [LING et al., 1970]. For recalcitrant and severe problems, one may employ methysergide (2 mg b.i.d. after meals) or ergonovine maleate (0.2 mg b.i.d. after meals), which is usually reserved for children over 10 years and particularly adolescents. These preparations are used rarely, and then for only a 3-month period followed by at least 1 month rest, because of the hazard of fibrotic disorders with methysergide [GRAHAM et al., 1966]. It is also wise to maintain these patients on phenobarbital or phenytoin at the same time.

It is usually unnecessary to go beyond the simple first order drugs. Phenobarbital or phenytoin adequately handle approximately 80% of patients. After 4–6 month control, medication may be withdrawn and reinstituted if symptoms recur.

In addition to pharmacotherapy, one must evaluate the life style and emotional state of the child, followed by appropriate advice. Referral for psychotherapy is occasionally necessary.

Prognosis

Migraine is a lifetime disorder, with a tendency to recur. Manifestations may differ somewhat at different ages and years can go by with only insignificant trouble. Childhood is not exempt, but manifestations differ. Attacks of headache are generally shorter, associated symptomatology such as nausea and vomiting may dominate the picture, and the classic visual prodromal symptoms are less marked. The syndromes of complicated migraine are more common in children than in adults and most have their onset in childhood, sometimes as early as 1–2 years of age.

References

BASSER, L.S.: Benign paroxysmal vertigo of childhood. Brain *87:* 141–152 (1964).
BICKERSTAFF, E.R.: Basilar artery migraine. Lancet *1:* 15–17 (1961).
BILLE, B.: Migraine in school children. Acta paediat. *51:* suppl. 136, pp. 1–151 (1962).
BLASS, J.P.; AVIGAN, J., and UHLENDORF, B.W.: A defect in pyruvate decarboxylase in a child with intermittent movement disorder. J. clin. Invest. *49:* 423–432 (1970).
BRUTON, C.J.; CORSELLIS, J.A.N., and RUSSELL, A.: Hereditary hyper-ammonemia. Brain *93:* 423–434 (1970).
CONNOR, R.C.R.: Complicated migraine. A study of permanent neurological and visual defects caused by migraine. Lancet *ii:* 1072–1075 (1962).
COUCH, J.R.; ZIEGLER, D.K., and HASSANEIN, R.: Amytriptyline in the prophylaxis of migraine. Neurology *26:* 121–127 (1976).
CULLEN, K.J., and MACDONALD, W.B.: The periodic syndrome, its nature and prevalence. Med. J. Aust. *ii:* 167–173 (1963).
DUNN, D.W., and SNYDER, C.H.: Benign paroxysmal vertigo of childhood. Am. J. Dis. Child. *130:* 1099–1100 (1976).
FENICHEL, G.M.: Migraine as a cause of benign paroxysmal vertigo in childhood. J. Pediat. *71:* 114–115 (1967).
FRIEDMAN, A.P.; HARTER, D.H., and MERRITT, H.H.: Ophthalmoplegic migraine. Archs. Neurol. *7:* 320–327 (1962).
GASCON, G., and BARLOW, C.: Juvenile migraine presenting as an acute confusional state. Pediatrics *45:* 628–635 (1970).
GOLDEN, G.S., and FRENCH, J.H.: Basilar artery migraine in young children. Pediatrics *56:* 722–726 (1975).
GRAHAM, J.R.; SUBY, H.I.; LECOMPTE, P.R., and SADOWSKY, N.L.: Fibrotic disorders associated with methysergide therapy for headache. New. Engl. J. Med. *274:* 359–368 (1966).
GREENBLATT, S.H.: Posttraumatic transient cerebral blindness. Association with migraine and seizure diathesis. J. Am. med. Ass. *225:* 1073–1076 (1973).
HAAS, D.C., and SOVNER, R.D.: Migraine attacks triggered by mild head trauma, and their relation to certain post-traumatic disorders in childhood. J. Neurol. Neurosurg. Psychiat. *32:* 548–554 (1969).
HAAS, D.C.; PINEDA, G., and LOURIE, H.: Juvenile head trauma syndromes and their relationship to migraine. Archs. Neurol. *32:* 730–737 (1975).
HAMMOND, J.: The late sequellae of recurrent vomiting of childhood. Dev. Med. Child. Neurol. *16:* 15–22 (1974).
HOLGUIN, J., and FENICHEL, G.M.: Migraine. J. Pediat. *70:* 290–297 (1967).
ISLER, W.: Acute hemiplegias and hemisyndromes in childhood. Clin. Dev. Med., vol. 41/42 (Lippincott, Philadelphia 1971).
KOENIGSBERGER, M.R.; CHUTORIAN, A.M.; GOLD, A.P., and SCHVEY, M.S.: Benign paroxysmal vertigo of childhood. Neurology *20:* 1108–1113 (1970).

Ling, W.; Oftedal, G., and Weinberg, W.: Depressive illness in childhood presenting as severe headache. Am. J. Dis. Child. *120:* 122–124 (1970).

Schwartz, I.H. and Lombroso, C.T.: 14 and 6/second positive spiking (ctenoids) in electroencephalogram of primary school pupils. J. Pediat. *72:* 678–682 (1968).

Verret, S. and Steele, J.C.: Alternating hemiplegia in childhood. A report of eight patients with complicated migraine beginning in infancy. Pediatrics *47:* 675–680 (1971).

Watson, P. and Steele, J.C.: Paroxysmal dysequilibrium in the migraine syndrome of childhood. Archs. Otolar. *99:* 177–179 (1974).

Weber, R.B. and Reinmuth, O.M.: The treatment of migraine with propranolol. Neurology *22:* 366–369 (1972).

Whitehouse, D.; Pappas, J.A.; Escala, P.H., and Livingston, S.: Electroencephalographic changes in children with migraine. New Engl. J. Med. *276:* 23–27 (1967).

Dr. Charles F. Barlow, Neurologist-in-Chief, Children's Hospital Medical Center, *Boston, MA 02115* (USA)

Autogenic Biofeedback Treatment for Migraine

STEVEN L. FAHRION

Department of Psychiatry and Psychology, Mayo Clinic, Rochester, Minn.

Contents

Introduction	47
Autogenic Biofeedback Training	48
Single Group Outcome Studies	50
Controlled Studies	56
Possible Mechanisms	59
Training Procedures	63
Conclusions	68
References	69

Introduction

The concept that the autonomic nervous system regulates the activity of the body only at an involuntary level, below the level of consciousness, is presently subject to debate. Evidence for learned control of autonomic functions is accumulating both with animals [DICARA and STONE, 1970; FIGAR, 1965; MILLER, 1969] and with humans [FOWLER and KIMMEL, 1962; KOPPMAN et al., 1974; TAUB and EMURIAN, 1976].

Autogenic training, a system of psychosomatic self-regulation which developed in Germany around the turn of the century, permits the gradual acquisition of autonomic control [SCHULTZ and LUTHE, 1969]. This control is not active; rather it develops out of a 'passive concentration' through which the trainee intends to move toward certain effects (e.g., relaxation) and yet remains detached as to his actual progress. The point of focus of his concentration is on visual, auditory, and somatic imagery that is employed to induce specific physiological changes such as hand warmth or muscle relaxation.

Biofeedback training is a rubric applied to a collection of techniques that may be useful in accelerating psychosomatic self-regulation. Physiological activity is monitored, and visual and auditory instruments are used to show the patient what is happening to normally unconscious bodily functions. Control of a wide variety of physiological parameters has been demonstrated, and seems limited only by the opportunity to continuously monitor the level of function in a physiological system, by the possibility of providing continuous feedback on that level, and by the expectations of success on the part of the patient [LEEB et al., 1976].

Autogenic Biofeedback Training

Autogenic biofeedback training [GREEN et al., 1975] represents an integration of the two above-mentioned self-regulatory techniques which has wide-ranging application in medicine, psychology, and education. One major focus of this form of training is voluntary control of sympathetic nervous system activation. Medical practitioners have long recognized that hand temperature declines during stress and increases with relaxation. Vasoconstriction during stress is part of an adaptive biological pattern that has the effect of preparing the body for 'fight or flight' by moving blood out of the periphery, into the deep muscles and up to the head [MITTLEMANN and WOLFF, 1939; ACKNER, 1956; BOUDEWYNS, 1976]. Vasoconstriction in the hands is primarily a function of sympathetic activation; thus, vasodilation is a one-variable index of decrease in sympathetic outflow, as the peripheral vasculature does not have significant parasympathetic innervation. Since skin temperature in the hands is directly related to peripheral blood flow, an increase in hand temperature is used as a convenient index in developing voluntary control of sympathetic activity [SARGENT et al., 1972].

Psychosomatic medicine has emphasized the importance of stress in inducing pathological dysfunction in patients. Autogenic biofeedback training (ABT) for hand warming produces changes opposite to those evoked by stress, and promotes healthy autonomic functioning. Thus, it is becoming a useful technique in preventative medicine, one such application being the prevention of migraine headaches.

Although it is commonly estimated that 5–10% of the US population suffers from migraine attacks, in three separate epidemiological surveys WATERS and O'CONNOR [1975] found the prevalence of migraine to be between 23 and 29% in women, and between 15 and 20% in men. Thus, 'migraine is much more prevalent than the frequently quoted figure of about 10% of the population, which does not seem to be based on any particular survey'.

Current treatment procedures for migraine typically have significant side effects that reduce patients' acceptance [ANTHONY and LANCE, 1972]. As SARGENT et al. [1973] have noted, 'for the most part, migraine attacks, although intensely disabling at times, are benign disorders for which patients are often overly medicated and are frequently given potentially addicting drugs'.

The pathophysiology of migraine remains poorly understood though it has been the subject of intensive scientific research over the past four decades. GRAHAM and WOLFF [1938] documented an increase in pulsation of the temporal artery during the headache phase, and showed that ergotamine tartrate decreased the amplitude of arterial pulsations while providing headache relief. (Previous work with histamine had clearly shown that stretched extracranial arteries were capable of producing pain.) Thus, the vascular theory of migraine developed in which migraine was seen as a dysfunction of cranial arteries, involving occlusive vasoconstriction of the cerebral arteries in the pre-headache phase, and dilation and distention primarily of branches of the external carotid arteries in the headache phase [SCHUMACHER and WOLFF, 1941]. That this dysfunction of vascular behavior in the head is related to intense sympathetic dysfunction is evident from the fact that cold hands typically accompany this syndrome. To emphasize, for the moment, this autonomic dysfunction, is not to minimize the importance of biochemical factors, which will be discussed below.

The ABT treatment of migraines did not, however, grow out of a theoretical consideration of the neural influences in migraine; rather, it developed as the result of a serendipitous observation. GREEN et al. [1975], in exploring the utility of combining autogenic techniques with thermal biofeedback, discovered that one of the housewives in their initial training group 'spontaneously' recovered from a migraine after about 15 min of practice of the technique in the lab. This recovery was accompanied by a sudden vasodilation in both hands and an increase in hand temperature of 5.5°C in 2 min. The researchers, observing the sudden change in hand temperature, asked the subject, 'What happened?' The subject replied, 'How did you know I lost my migraine?' [GREEN et al., 1975]. Two additional migraineurs were then trained, with positive results. After 2 weeks of practice with the meter and phrases, the first of these subjects stopped taking drugs and has remained free of migraine to the present, about 8 years.

Single Group Outcome Studies

Subsequently, SARGENT, an internist at the Menninger Foundation, initiated a single group outcome study of the effect of ABT in migraine control [SARGENT et al., 1973]. Their report concerns the treatment of 75 subjects who were either self-referred or referred by physicians in the community. Careful attention was paid to diagnosis; each patient had a detailed history, complete physical examination, and laboratory studies including EEG, skull X-rays, echoencephalogram, chest X-ray, serology, CBC, and urinalysis. Subjects with severe psychologic and/or physical disorders were eliminated from the study. Of the 75 subjects, 57 had migraine headaches, 11 had tension headaches, and 5 had combined headaches, and there were 2 with cluster headaches. Training followed basic procedures to be described below. Headache ratings were made over a 1-month baseline prior to treatment, as well as throughout the course of training and the follow-up periods.

Approximately 81% of the migraine patients followed for over 150 days were helped to a significant extent. The degree of improvement ranged from slight to very good (table I). The remaining 19% of the migraine patients showed little or no reduction of headache activity and drug use. It may be of interest with regard to the latter that the criteria of training success with these patients was merely a one degree net increase within a 5- to 15- min trial. No *absolute level criterion* was used, such as the one suggested below.

In a more recent, unpublished summary of 5 years of pilot work with 110 migrainous patients, SARGENT [1975] reported that 36 did not complete the training and follow-up for various reasons, for an attrition rate of 33%. The remaining 74 patients were categorized as to percent of headache reduction with the following results (table II). When only those patients falling in the moderate to very good improvement categories were considered to be significantly improved, 55 patients or 74% of those completing training fell in this category.

In another unpublished study conducted at the Menninger Foundation, PEARSE et al. [1974] evaluated an innovative program designed to reduce the duration of training. Headache patients in this study were subjected to the same diagnostic battery described above, and then were given intensive autogenic biofeedback training (a 1- to 2-hour training session daily for 5 consecutive days). Records were kept concerning headache frequency, severity, duration, degree of disability, medications used, the patient's ability to feel warmth in the hands, the speed with which he was able to feel

Table I. Degree and type of improvement for 42 migraine headache patients

Degree of improvement	Type of improvement	Number of migraine patients	
None	headache activity continued at the same level with little or no reduction in medication	8	19% not improved
Slight	shortened headache duration, for instance, from 24 to 12 h reduced severity of headache, for instance, from severe to moderate, and reduced frequency of headache, for instance, from 20 headache days/mo. to 15/mo.	9	
Moderate	all in the slight category and, in addition, aborting headache after its onset by voluntarily relaxing, and some reduction of drug use	9	
Good	all in the slight and moderate categories and, in addition, detection of *preheadache* symptoms and voluntarily relaxing to avoid headache, and considerable reduction of drug use	10	81% improved
Very good	all in the slight, moderate and good categories, and, in addition, complete elimination of drug use for headache relief except for a few brief, isolated episodes	6	
Total		42	

Table II. Categories of improvement for 74 patients completing 270 days of training and follow-up

Percent reduction	Categories of improvement	Number of patients
0–9	'no improvement'	12
10–25	'slight improvement'	7
26–50	'Moderate improvement'	22
51–75	'Good improvement'	16
76–100	'Very good improvement'	17
		74

hand warming sensations, the degree of relaxation achieved, temperatures recorded at the beginning and conclusion of each practice session, and the patient's ability to control his headaches with the use of the ABT exercises. Additional procedures used included neck and shoulder exercises to loosen stiff muscles, diaphragmatic breathing exercises to encourage relaxation, periodic scanning of the body for early detection of increase in tension, and encouragement of the patient to diminish the habitual use of drugs for headache relief as soon as training goals were reached.

A detailed follow-up questionnaire was sent to each of the 40 patients in the study 12 months following training. 27 or 67.5% returned the questionnaires. Of these, 21 were female and 6 were male. Data for 3 females and 1 male had to be dropped because of incorrect completion of the questionnaire. Subjects ranged in age from 14 to 71 years, and were primarily of the middle to upper middle economic income groups.

Subjects were asked to rate themselves on each of the above seven categories as either *much better* (+2), *some better* (+1), *about the same* (0), *some worse* (-1), or *much worse* (-2). Thus, each subject could receive a score ranging from +14 to -14.

Table III depicts the results. Success in managing headache behavior was experienced by 82.6% of the subjects with 17.4% remaining unchanged, and with no one ranking in the somewhat worse or considerably worse categories. The modal improvement score equaled +14; the median improvement score equaled +12.5. Table IV illustrates the drug reduction that was possible for these patients. 55% were able to achieve a reduction in headache medications of between 76 and 100% while 20% showed no reduction at all. Average reduction in medication was 80%.

The results also show a significant positive relationship between the ability to relax and headache improvement, as well as between drug reduction and headache improvement. Finally, there was a significant positive relationship between the ability to achieve deeper levels of relaxation and the ability to reduce drug intake.

Overall the study is of interest both as a replication of the previous work of SARGENT *et al.*, and as an extension, in that the short-term intensive format seems equally beneficial in comparison to longer term ABT programs.

The Menninger results have also been replicated by other investigators. In presenting a clinical series of 58 headache patients treated with biofeedback over a 5-year period, ADLER and ADLER [1976] report that in 86% of the patients, there was an overall apparent cure or major alleviation of symptoms (less than 25% of original headache frequency) and a concomitant reduction of drug use. In the 1- to 5-year follow-up, the results were essentially the same as at the end of treatment, with the greatest success rate for tension headache (88%), then migraine (81%), then mixed tension/migraine and cluster headaches (both 60%). (The standard biofeedback

Table III. Distribution of headache improvement scores for 23 patients completing a 1-year follow-up questionnaire[1]

Category	Number of Ss	Average score	% of Ss
Considerably better (+ 9 to + 14)	17	+ 12.5	73.9
Somewhat better (+ 3 to + 8)	2	+ 7.0	8.7
Unchanged (− 2 to + 2)	4	0	17.4
Somewhat worse (− 8 to − 3)	0	0	0
Considerably worse	0	0	0

[1] Adapted from PEARSE *et al.* [1974].

Table IV. Distribution of drug reduction scores for 20 patients[1]

Degree of drug reduction	Number of Ss	% of Ss	Average drug reduction, %
Very good (76–100%)	11	55	87.5
Good (51–75%)	3	15	72.3
Moderate (26–50%)	2	10	50.0
Slight (11–25%)	0	0	—
None (0–10%)	4	20	0.0

[1] Adapted from PEARSE *et al.* [1974].

treatment procedure for tension headaches is not ABT; rather, it involves feeding back to the patient an index of the level of frontalis muscle tension [BUDZYNSKI *et al.*, 1970]. With the help of the feedback the patient learns to recognize the internal cues that go with reduction of muscle tension in those muscle groups that are primarily activated in tension headache.) Since, as FRIEDMAN [1964] has noted, 'ninety percent of chronic headaches are vascular headaches of the migraine type, muscle contraction headaches, or combinations of the two types', these results suggest wide applicability of biofeedback training procedures in the treatment of headache.

The results with 21 headache patients treated in the Mayo Clinic will be presented here for the first time. These patients represent all those diagnosed migraine and migraine/tension patients who completed the training program and for whom at least 6-month follow-up data could be obtained. (Such data was unavailable for two additional patients.) In every case diagnosis was established by a neurologist facilitated by EEG, skull X-ray, computerized-axial tomography scanning and other medical procedures necessary to rule out the presence of organicity. No patients were eliminated from the remaining group on the basis of psychological or physical disorders other than migraine. Of the 21 patients, 11 had migraine headaches and 10 had combined migraine and tension headaches. All patients had had chemotherapy prior to beginning biofeedback, and many had had physical therapy. 17 of the 21 patients had had significant headache problems for more than a decade (several for 30–40 years,) and the remainder had had headaches for several years.

Training followed procedures described below, with 8 of the patients receiving intensive training. Headache ratings and medication records were obtained throughout the treatment period and for several months post-treatment. Patients have been followed for 6–13 months (average = 10.1 months).

Two independent raters categorized these patients with 95.2% agreement: the more conservative placement is presented in table V. Approximately 71.5% of the patients were helped to a significant extent according to the follow-up data, the improvement ranging from slight to very good. Although caution must be taken in comparing results due to the small sample sizes and possible differences in the populations sampled, these results appear to differ from those obtained at Menninger's in two ways. First, the percentage of patients in the 'very good' category is much higher. It is hypothesized that this has to do with improvements in training procedures since they were initially developed, including this investigator's insistence upon the attainment of high absolute hand temperatures as a criterion of training success. Further research will be required to explore the importance of adherence to this criterion. It should be noted that some patients in the 'very good' category have improved sufficiently to be able to dispense entirely with practice without recurrence of their symptoms.

The second difference concerns the addition of the 'not sustained' category which includes 23.8% of the patients. This category probably includes patients who would have been likely to fall into the attrition group in the Menninger research. A retrospective review of the 6 cases showing lack of sustained improvement (including the one showing no improvement), revealed that 2 patients had vocational stresses that prevented them from taking the time to practice, despite good initial improvement. After train-

Table V. Degree and type of improvement for 21 migraine and migraine/tension headache patients

Degree of improvement	Type of improvement	Number of migraine patients	
None	headache activity continued at the same level with little or no reduction in medication	1	28.6% not improved
Not sustained	initial improvement followed by regression to no improvement, where practice was discontinued or substantially reduced	5	
Slight	shortened headache duration, for instance, from 24 to 12 h reduced severity of headache, for instance, from 20 headache days/mo. 15/mo.	3	
Moderate	all in the slight category and, in addition, aborting headache after its onset by voluntarily relaxing, and some reduction of drug use	1	71.4% improved
Good	all in the slight and moderate categories and, in addition, detection of *preheadache* symptoms and voluntarily relaxing to avoid headache, and considerable reduction of drug use	1	
Very good	all in the slight, moderate and good categories, and, in addition, complete elimination of drug use for headache relief except for a few brief, isolated episodes	10	
Total		21	

ing, one of these patients had gone the longest period in 10 years without a headache, but then markedly expanded her business efforts. One patient showed definite evidence of drug dependence, and though she had been able to reduce medication during and for 2 months following treatment, upon follow-up she had returned to her previous pattern of usage. 2 patients showed probable placebo response. One of these had had headaches for 31 years prior to treatment, with 69 days of hospitalization in the previous year for headache treatment. Over the years she had had 61 (!) different medications for her headaches, as well as physical and psychiatric therapies. Following ABT she began to be able to abort her migraines, and 2 months later she wrote, 'I feel like a new person. I had become very despondent and moody. I had lost all interest in everything, and it was an effort just to live from day to day. I lived in constant fear of another headache... It is a great feeling to be able to relax my whole body. I've got a whole new outlook on life. My disposition is so much better and I feel happy. Things don't upset me and bother me like they did, and I don't have to worry a headache is going to make me cancel plans. My daughters say they've got a new mother. I am very thankful for the training.' Later on that same month she had a headache she could not abort without medication, which she seemed reluctant to take. From that point on, she had increasing difficulty, with regression to about her previous level of headache activity a year later. No apparent reason could be found for the lack of improvement in the final patient.

Children seem to learn voluntary control of hand warmth even more quickly than adults, with beneficial effects on their migraines [PEPER and GROSSMAN, 1974]. One clinical series of 32 patients between 9 and 18 years old showed poor results with only 2 patients, both of whom displayed substantial depression [DIAMOND and FRANKLIN, 1976]. These investigators concluded that biofeedback is an excellent tool in treating childhood migraine.

Controlled Studies

Well-designed, controlled studies of biofeedback treatment procedures such as ABT present special problems in comparison to studies designed to evaluate medication effects. Theoretically it should be possible to compare the effects of biofeedback training with those induced by an 'attention-placebo' condition. Examples of presumably suitable attention placebo conditions include a false feedback (i.e., noncontingent feedback) treatment, biofeedback training on a supposedly nonrelevant physiological modality (e.g., training migraine patients to increase brain rhythm frequency, while, of course, promoting an expectation of success), or training on a relevant modality but in the opposite direction (e.g., toward hand *cooling*). Practically speaking, each of these approaches presents problems as a control for the hand warming procedure. Patients quickly learn to recognize false feedback, particularly of muscle tension but also of hand warmth. Certainly this recognition will occur before the conclusion of the 6–10 sessions required for completion of training, with deleterious effects on the motivation of control group members. Secondly, it is difficult to find truly nonrelevant training modalities which have face validity and invoke patient acceptance. One investigator attempted to train migraine patients for increased brain rhythm frequencies as a control condition, only to discover that his subjects would not tolerate the subjective sensations of tension and jitteriness that accompanied this training. Thirdly, by now, many migraine patients are aware of a presumed relationship between hand warming and headache relief, and it is difficult to mobilize an expectation of success on their part when they are given training for hand cooling. Development of an effective double-blind design for a biofeedback modality such as hand temperature, where the subjective effects are easily noted, presents even more formidable problems. (The double-blind study of biofeedback brain rhythm training, for example, is less difficult.)

To these difficulties must be added the fact that effective training depends on an open warm rapport between trainer and trainee. Great differences in the individual effectiveness of trainers have been noted in the literature, and attempts to force the delivery of training into a narrow definition of standardization inevitably results in a decrement in a subject's ability to learn hand warming. Despite these difficulties and the newness of this treatment approach, a few controlled studies exist. Nonetheless, a definitive evaluation of the usefulness of this technique will not be evident for several years. The most notable effort in this regard is the federally funded study currently in progress at the Menninger Foundation under the direction of Dr. JOSEPH SARGENT; the results should be available in approximately 3 years.

WICKRAMASKERA [1973] reported on the treatment of 2 migraine patients using a multiple baseline design across behaviors [KAZDIN, 1973]. These patients were first treated (unsuccessfully) with frontalis muscle biofeedback, and then later with thermal biofeedback with a positive response. Both had had migraines for approximately 30 years, had received psychotherapy and chemotherapy, and had been examined and treated at leading medical clinics, all without positive outcome. Both had become quite resentful and skeptical, particularly after the unsuccessful muscle biofeedback treatment. After 16 and 18 sessions of muscle biofeedback (respectively) they showed only slight reduction in intensity of headache and no decline in frequency. Another 5 week baseline period provided data on headache frequency and intensity, and temperature training was begun. The hand warming skill was acquired more quickly than had been the case with frontalis relaxation. The frequency and intensity of headaches declined as these 2 patients increased their skill in hand warming. While analgesic consumption did not change during baseline and training periods, at 3-month follow-up both patients reported that they had reduced their consumption to an occasional aspirin for non-headache related events. These results support the idea that temperature training is causally related to reduction of migraine, rather than simply mobilizing placebo-suggestion effects.

Drury et al. [1975] used a multiple baseline design to examine the effectiveness of ABT in the treatment of migraine. Patients were referred by cooperating neurologists and additionally screened for migraine using the criteria of Wolff [1963]. Baseline measures included hourly ratings of headache intensity, as well as frequency and type of medication used. Treatment was introduced only after a reliable baseline was obtained. The treatment (ABT) was introduced to individual patients sequentially, in such a way that the effect of treatment was observed in the headache and medication records of one patient before treatment was introduced to the next patient. The results indicated that the treatment package was functionally related to reduction in headache activity and recorded medication usage.

Turin and Johnson [1976] trained 7 migraineurs in finger warming without the aid of the autogenic training phrases. To control for placebo-expectancy efforts, 3 of the 7 subjects were trained in finger cooling prior to warming. Despite these subjects' positive expectations that cooling would be therapeutic, their headache level either remained at baseline levels or increased. When subjects were trained to warm, migraine activity was reduced significantly. These results again indicate that the efficacy of hand warming is independent of suggestion effects. This conclusion also seems plausible in view of the fact that placebo medications typically produce improvement in 5–25% of the patients, while in the single group outcome studies reviewed above 70–80% of the patients showed significant improvement.

Zamani [1975] in a related biofeedback migraine treatment approach taught one group of patients to constrict the extracranial temporal artery with pulse amplitude feedback, while using as a control a deep muscle relaxation training regime with a second group. The biofeedback group changed significantly in terms of headache duration, frequency, and medication usage. In contrast, the relaxation group showed no statistically significant decrease in any of these variables.

Two successful cases in the Mayo series essentially represent inadvertently controlled single case experiments following an ABAB design [Barlow and Hersen, 1973]. These cases also illustrate some of the difficulties in evaluating longer term results with this treatment.

ABT was begun with a 43-year-old farmer after he had required excessive doses of morphine to alleviate headache pain, with deleterious effects on excretory functions. He had migraines since he was 10 years old, which had become worse in the previous 7 years, with 1–2 headaches per week and severe headaches requiring injections every 2 weeks. Headaches typically began during sleep in the right frontotemporal region, then spread to the left side as well, and usually lasted 1½–2 days. Photophobia was common, but nausea and vomiting occurred only occasionally. Initial hand temperatures were in the low 80s (°F). By the end of an intensive week of training (8 sessions) he was able to warm to 95.4°F while sitting up with his eyes open. At the midpoint of the training week he was able to abort two headaches without medication. 1 month later, he had continued to be headache-free; an attack had begun on several occasions but he had been able to abort each one. Shortly thereafter he visited his local medical doctor who scoffed at his relaxation practice, undermining his confidence. 2 months following training he was still doing fairly well, although he was requiring some medication. At 4 months follow-up, he reported that he had had a total of 2½ months with no headaches at all, and then they started coming back. Further inquiry revealed that this relapse was associated with more sporadic, less motivated practice. He had been discouraged as well by an article suggesting that biofeedback would not help headaches associated with depression. A return to practice was urged. When he returned for a 1-year follow-up, he reported that following an increase in his practice, his headaches had gradually decreased in frequency, with no headache in the previous 3 months. He had gradually reduced his medication and had not required analgesics for 5 months. A more relaxed approach to life had also been noted by the patient.

Another patient who experienced a recurrence of headache associated with discontinuance of practice was a 35-year-old woman initially referred for treatment of intractable migraines of the classical type. She had had migraines for 10 years and was having headaches 5–7 days per week, and consuming 6–7 doses of cafergot P-B per headache day. Initial hand temperatures were in the 70s and low 80s (°F) and she quickly learned to warm to mid 90s. By her 4th week of training she had had one 7-day headache-free period. Treatment was discontinued, and she continued home practice resulting in several additional headache-free weeks. She then stopped her practice and at 2 month follow-up reported that she had had 2 headaches, one of them quite severe. She had additional academic pressures over the next 3 weeks, further reducing her practice and exacerbating her headaches. Then she began more intensive practice and improved so much that when, 3 months later, she had to face the stresses of major surgery, she had no headaches whatsoever, nor have they returned in a subsequent 3-month period.

Possible Mechanisms

There seems little doubt that emotional factors are of prime significance in the etiology of muscle contraction headache, although no single psychological dynamic can account for their onset [MARTIN *et al.,* 1967]. The existence of 'migraine personality' is a matter of some debate, though the exploration of this topic is beyond the scope of this article. Clinicians will recognize, however, that from a psychological standpoint, the kind of relaxed detachment that is required to facilitate hand warming is quite the opposite of the state that normally precedes the migraine attack.

Physiologically, migraineurs tend to display high vasomotor reactivity. BURCH et al. [1942] reported that subjects who showed small and limited spontaneous peripheral vasomotor activity could generally be described as placid and emotionally stable, and as readily adjusting to the experimental situation. On the other hand, those who demonstrated large fluctuations were more emotional, inquisitive and anxious. It is possible to detect and reliably quantify individual differences in autonomic lability [LACEY and LACEY, 1958], and such quantification may provide a useful tool in exploring the mechanisms underlying ABT treatment of migraines. As STERN [1966] has hypothesized, the greater the spontaneous lability of a physiological response system, such as peripheral vasomotor activity, the more easily that system can be conditioned by environmental stimuli including life stresses. Therefore, it is likely that a high level of spontaneous activity in a given physiological system is associated with an increased probability of developing abnormal functioning in that system.

It may be of interest in this regard that the incidence of migraine tends to decline with age, as does the amount of spontaneous fluctuation in various physiological systems. Furthermore, DALESSIO [1963] described a series of studies of the vascular effects of methysergide which suggested that this medication has its effects by dampening vascular instability. Unless some such therapeutic mechanism is involved it is difficult to explain how agents which increase vasocontriction (e.g., ergotamine tartrate), those inducing no evident vasomotor effects (e.g., methysergide), and those which have vasodilator effects (e.g., ABT) could all have beneficial effects on migraine headaches. What these agents may share is a stabilizing effect on vasomotor tone.

While the functioning of the sympathetic vasodilator system is complex and not yet fully understood, it is basically under the control of the limbic-hypothalmic axis. Much also remains to be learned about the mechanisms involved in the development of voluntary control, but the basic sequence of events would seem to be as follows: peripheral somatic activity is perceived, first with the aid of the biofeedback instrument, and then through internal cueing → limbic response → hypothalmic response → autonomic response → peripheral somatic response. Thus, a cybernetic loop is created which permits an alteration of the homeostatic level of functioning. As SARGENT et al. [1973] have noted, 'since the sympathetic control centers for vascular behavior are located in subcortical structures, it seems that the (ABT) attack on vascular dysfunction in the head is linked to a general relaxation of sympathetic outflow rather than through hydraulic maneuvering of blood in various portions of the body'. In support of this point, PRICE and TURSKEY [1976] found high positive correlations between blood volume changes in the hand and extracranial arteries.

The place of biochemical factors in the pathophysiology of migraine is a topic of intensive investigation. Several lines of evidence suggest that serotonin may play a role in the migraine syndrome, and the action of catecholamines, histamine, and kinins has also been studied in relation to these headaches. Serotonin is known to have a differential effect on blood vessels, inducing constriction of large arteries and veins, and dilation of arterioles and capillaries [ANTHONY and LANCE, 1972]. Thus, decreased levels of circulating serotonin could be responsible for both the dilation of scalp arteries and the skin pallor (due to capillary constriction) seen during the headache phase.

APPENZELLER [1969] advanced a bipartite hypothesis concerning the mechanism of migraine. According to this hypothesis, vessels that are (1) tonically contracted, due to the excessive sympathetic effects, dilate due to (2) the activity of vasoactive substances (e.g., serotonin, hormones, monosodium 1-glutamate). The rapid change in size of the extracranial vessels is painful. This hypothesis suggests that *either* reduction of sympathetic activity or administration of internal vasodilator substances (or both) should be helpful.

Biofeedback clearly has a role in reducing sympathetic activation. In addition, albeit a speculative hypothesis, the possibility that ABT may also have certain biochemical effects will have to be ruled out before a full understanding of the mechanisms underlying this treatment can be realized. Alteration in the level of biochemical factors associated with controlled physiological events has already been demonstrated in animals. DICARA and STONE [1970] showed that rats taught biofeedback-induced increases in heart rate showed significantly higher cardiac and brain stem catecholamine levels than those trained to decrease heart rate. Yoked controls receiving noncontingent feedback showed no such changes. No studies of the effect of ABT on serum levels of serotonin and various other biochemicals under scrutiny as to their role in migraine have, as yet, been conducted. Until the possibility of such effects has been ruled out, it should be apparent that acceptance of the usefulness of this form of treatment does not require acceptance of the 'dry theory' of migraine, the hypothesis that headache pain arises simply from stretched walls of dilated vessels following neurogenic decrease in vascular tone. Rather, it seems possible that the hand warming procedure may also influence the lowered pain threshold and humorally mediated inflammation of the vessel wall [SICUTERI, 1972]; otherwise it may be difficult to account for the ability of trained patients to abort the headache after its onset.

While the testing of this hypothesis and an exploration of the mechanisms underlying this form of treatment will await the requisite research studies, ABT seems to belie the argument that the etiological mechanisms must be known before a prevention or treatment approach can be developed. In this perspective, ABT is pragmatic and symptom-focused, betraying its relationship to other behavioral or 'learning' treatment approaches, in contrast to psychotherapy. Nonetheless, as the underlying mechanism becomes known, it seems likely that we may be able to further increase the effectiveness of ABT through a refinement of our biofeedback training procedures.

Development of voluntary control of temporal artery diameter through direct biofeedback training might be useful, for example, for patients who do not improve from ABT alone. SARGENT *et al.* [1973] showed a considerable decoupling of hand temperature and frontotemporal skin temperature changes with only small changes occurring in the latter. ENGEL and SCHAEFER [1974] demonstrated both the possiblity and the relative difficulty of learning voluntary control of forehead temperatures, probably because of the greater dependence of the head on core temperature. KOPPMAN *et al.* [1974] and SAVILL and KOPPMAN [1975] successfully taught subjects to dilate and constrict the temporal artery using pulse amplitude biofeedback. While this approach provides only a relative measure that varies from session to session, and has other characteristics such as difficulty in acquisition that probably make it a less desirable modality for basic training, its use as an *adjunct* to ABT should be thoroughly explored. It seems unlikely that such training will have the impact on general relaxation that ABT does since, as TAUB and EMURIAN [1976] have shown, the better a person is able to control skin temperature of a particular site through biofeedback alone, the more specific is the response to the trained portion of the body. ABT does not seem to have such localized effects. Even well-trained subjects continue to report warming in both hands and feet at the same time.

Finally, experienced autogenic trainers mention the phenomenon of autogenic shift – a fairly dramatic shift to a more relaxed response to the world in general – in well-trained ABT patients. The Cannon-Bard theory of emotion postulates two distinct aspects of emotion: (1) an upward discharge from the hypothalamus to the cortex that provides affective tone to sensations, thoughts and memories, and (2) a downward discharge from the hypothalamus to the viscera and skeletal muscles that produces the observable emotional expression. Thus, if indices of the latter are reduced through biofeedback training, it should be no surprise if a concomitant reduction in tonic cortical hyperactivation should also occur in the course of time.

Training Procedures

While there is some variability in the procedures used by various practitioners in teaching voluntary control of autonomic processes, those which are described here are fairly typical. Prior to beginning biofeedback training each potential trainee should have a medical workup to establish the diagnosis of vascular or tension-vascular headache. These workups are carefully reviewed by the trainer before he sees the patient; thus, a minimum amount of time is required for intake and diagnosis when the patient arrives for training.

The first 15–20 min of the initial appointment are spent developing rapport with the trainee and introducing the concept of biofeedback training. Particular emphasis is placed on explaining how biofeedback is applied to the trainee's specific disorder; that is, what body functions are being measured and how the normalization of these functions can help to alleviate the symptoms. The trainee is shown several graphs of successful training programs of other individuals with the intent of inducing a sense of hopefulness and positive expectancy about the treatment process. Migraine sufferers referred for training have typically undergone a variety of different treatments without successful results, and often feel somewhat hopeless or skeptical about the prospects of improving their condition.

The trainer also informs the client that positive results are likely, provided that two criteria are met: (1) the trainee must perform hand-warming exercises every day and must be able to sustain a hand temperature of at least 95.5°F for 10 min at a time; and (2) he should be able to increase hand temperature at a rate of at least 1°F/min. (These criteria are perhaps somewhat more stringent than those currently required by most biofeedback practitioners, but the maintenance of these criteria is considered to be important if the best clinical results are to be obtained.)

During the first appointment the trainee is monitored for baseline levels of skin temperature and frontalis EMG. The EMG baseline data is especially important for individuals with mixed migraine and tension headaches. Since the initial training is usually performed with the patient lying down, the initial baseline data is also taken in this position. Each physiological function is monitored over a 3-min period, with successive averaged readings taken every 20 sec with a digital integrator.

Many trainers site the skin temperature sensor on the first phalanx of the middle finger of the nondominant hand. The author prefers the placement on the first phalanx of the little finger of the nondominant hand, since it has been observed that the little finger is the most sensitive to autonomic arousal mechanisms (it both warms first and cools first), and the nondominant hand usually warms more rapidly than the dominant. This placement point is used for both baseline evaluation and for training.

As soon as baseline data is taken, the trainee is oriented to the training process, with remarks such as the following: 'At this point I'm going to give you some autogenic training phrases and I want you to say each phrase over and over to yourself. Your attitude as you do this is quite important. This is the kind of thing where the more you try and relax, the less it will happen. So the best approach is to have the intention to warm and to relax, but to remain detached about your actual results. Since everyone can learn voluntary control of these processes, I would surmise it is just a matter of time until you do, and therefore you can afford to be detached about the results. Secondly, saying the phrases is good because it keeps them in mind, but it is not enough. The part of the brain that controls these processes doesn't understand language so it is important to translate the content of the phrase into some kind of an image. One of the phrases is, "my hands are heavy and warm". If you can actually imagine what it would feel like if your hands did feel heavy or if they did feel warm, that helps to bring on the changes. Or use a visual image; imagine you are lying out on the beach in the sun, or that you're holding hands over a campfire. Whatever works for you as a relaxing image that's the thing to use, but the imaging itself is important. Finally, if you simply trust your body to do what you're asking it to do then you will discover that it will.'

The modified autogenic training phrases developed by the Menninger Foundation Voluntary Controls Project (fig. 1) are then administered for approximately 20 min. During the first training session, only verbal feedback is given, because direct instrument feedback commonly induces performance anxiety on the part of the trainee at this stage. Therefore, the trainer observes

> I feel quite quiet... I am beginning to feel quite relaxed... My feet feel heavy and relaxed... My ankles, my knees, and my hips, feel heavy, relaxed, and comfortable... My solar plexus, and the whole central portion of my body, feel relaxed and quiet... My hands, my arms, and my shoulders, feel heavy, relaxed, and comfortable... My neck, my jaws, and my forehead feel relaxed... They feel comfortable and smooth... My whole body feels quiet, heavy, comfortable and relaxed.
>
> I am quite relaxed... My arms and hands are heavy and warm... I feel quite quiet... My whole body is relaxed and my hands are warm, relaxed and warm... My hands are warm... Warmth is flowing into my hands, they are warm... warm.

Fig. 1. Autogenic phrases.

the physiological response on the instrument and provides verbal feedback for improvement in hand temperature between each autogenic training phrase. The trainee might be told, 'You are beginning to get warmer', and 'You're now warming more rapidly', as these events occur. At each stage, the trainee is given encouragement and reinforcement; initially verbal feedback is not given when temperature decreases. Each time the trainee's hand temperature rises by 0.1°F he is informed that this has occurred. If his temperature is increasing rapidly, he will be told, 'You've gone up 0.3, 0.5, 1°F', and so forth. It has been observed that some trainees experience very rapid increases in hand temperature, up to 3–4°F/min.

During the first training session it is especially important that the autogenic training phrases be carefully paced to correspond with the trainee's actual physiological changes. If it appears that he is receiving special benefit from a particular phrase, no new phrase will be introduced for a period, and he will be allowed to continue with that phrase until the rate of temperature increase begins to slow down, at which point the next phrase will be introduced. If it appears that a phrase is not producing the desired response, a new phrase will be introduced sooner than usual, or that phrase might be repeated. It is important for the trainee to be given sufficient time between phrases to be able to repeat each phrase slowly at least three times.

Toward the end of the first session, auditory feedback will be introduced. Various instruments provide different forms of feedback, but the most widely used is a tone which decreases in pitch as the hands warm. Another sensitive and useful form of feedback is a tone which increases in pitch as the *rate* of warming increases.

Should a trainee show a temperature decline the trainer might say, 'There's been a slight temperature decrease, and there is nothing to do but to wait. Then it will turn around and you will begin to warm again.'

At the conclusion of the first training period, the trainee is asked to open his eyes and the remainder of the session is devoted to discussion of the experience, unhooking the instruments and assigning homework exercises.

Subsequent training sessions generally follow the same course as the first session, with baseline data taken at the beginning of each session. A typical appointment lasts an hour and consists of 20 min of training and 40 min of discussion. During the course of therapy, a variety of factors arise which the trainee wishes to discuss, e.g., the nature of his symptoms, past events relating to these symptoms, changes which are occurring as a result of therapy and so forth. It is considered important that the trainee and trainer develop an empathic relationship, so that the trainee feels the therapist is genuinely interested and willing to listen to any problems or issues he wishes to bring up. This discussion must be kept within reason, however, and not be allowed to generate excessive distraction from training.

In the case of individuals with tension headaches or mixed tension/migraine headaches, an alternative procedure is used. During the first two sessions, EMG activity is monitored while the trainee performs temperature training with the autogenic phrases. If there is a high correlation between temperature increase and EMG decrease during these sessions, temperature training is continued as a sole feedback modality. If not, training is divided between temperature and EMG, with temperature training performed first. During the initial stages of EMG training, verbal feedback is used, and audiofeedback is gradually introduced at low volume. No phrases or other special procedures are used during EMG training; the trainee is simply permitted to use the audiofeedback to inform himself of his progress toward relaxed levels.

After each session, the therapist makes a graph of the trainee's progress during that session, using the information taken down from the instruments during the training period. At the point where it is clear that he is beginning to show progress in training, these graphs are shown to the trainee, since they serve to reinforce a sense of accomplishment. Figure 2 illustrates the complete course of temperature training with a 43-year-old man referred for general relaxation training in relation to a variety of stress-related problems.

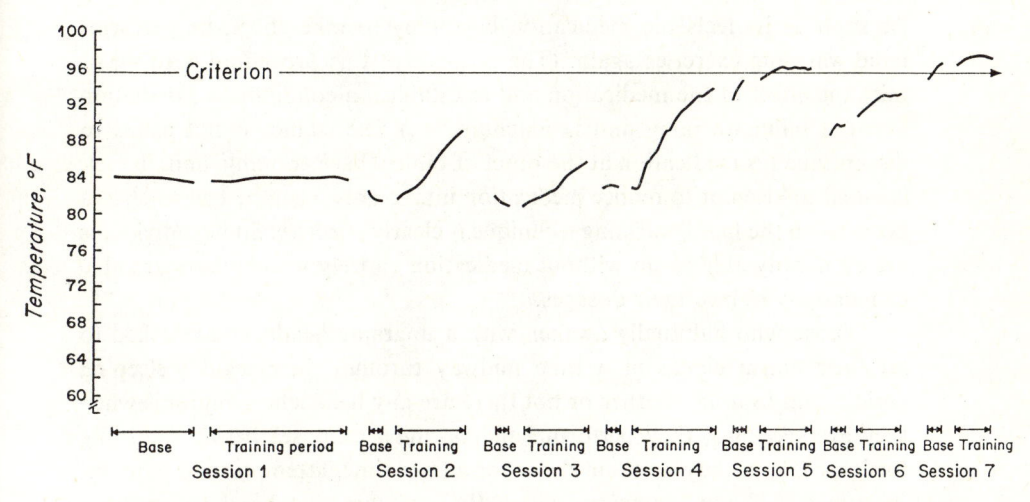

Fig. 2. Hand temperature in a 43-year-old man undergoing autogenic biofeedback training.

Some attention must be paid toward integrating the results of practice into the daily life of the trainee. Homework practice is considered imperative in facilitating a generalization of training skills. At the end of the first session, each individual being treated for headache is given a daily rating to chart headache activity hourly. The material from these sheets is subsequently averaged on a weekly basis and presented on a graph for the trainee's review. He is also given cassette tapes of the autogenic phrases, which he is instructed to take home and practice as often as possible, but at least once a day. As soon as he begins to demonstrate a capacity for temperature self-regulation, he is given an inexpensive monitoring device for home use. Hand temperature is recorded at the beginning and at the end of each homework practice session, and these results are reviewed by the trainer each week.

To facilitate generalization the trainee moves to a sittingup position as the sessions progress, first, with eyes closed, and then with eyes open. In addition to performing homework relaxation exercises, the trainee is asked to perform a mental scan of his body at various intervals of the day to note any tension that may be present, and to spend a few moments relaxing.

When a trainee begins to experience the onset of a headache, he is encouraged to spend 1–2 min performing hand-warming exercises before taking any medication. If he still feels the need for medication, he takes it.

As soon as he feels the medication beginning to take effect, he performs hand-warming exercises again. (The purpose of this procedure is to maximize the effect of the medication and to establish a conditioned association between hand warming and headache relief.) The trainee is not asked to discontinue his medication at the onset of biofeedback training, and, in fact, is asked to attempt to reduce medication intake only when he has reached a point when the hand-warming technique is clearly effective. Some individuals are eventually able to do without medication entirely while others are able to markedly reduce their dosages.

Those who habitually awaken with a migraine headache are asked to set their alarm clocks at a time midway through their regular sleeping period, and to note whether or not there are any headache symptoms when they awake. If so, they perform hand-warming exercises before returning to sleep. If not, they set their alarm for a later time, attempting to pinpoint the time when the symptoms occur. (It is known that hand temperature varies considerably during dream periods, and it is considered possible that dream content may be a source of many headache symptoms which originate during sleep.)

The final session includes a discussion of training progress achieved thus far, as well as orientation toward what remains to be done. The patient is instructed to attempt to maintain a hand temperature of 95.5°F for at least 10 min each day. The maintenance of deep, autonomic relaxation associated with high hand temperature is the factor which most effectively protects the individual from migraine attacks, by helping to establish a more normal psychophysiological posture. The trainee also continues to send the therapist headache report cards for the next few months. If it appears from these headache reports that he is experiencing difficulties, or if he does not send in the cards, the therapist telephones him to inquire about his progress, and to recommend whatever modifications in training methodology seem appropriate. As a routine procedure, the therapist telephones each trainee after several months for follow-up evaluation.

Conclusions

Autogenic biofeedback training (ABT) appears to be a promising technique for the treatment of migraine headaches. Relevant literature has been reviewed and some additional data presented along with speculations concerning possible mechanisms underlying this form of treatment. ABT exemplifies an important trend in psychosomatic medicine in shifting a major portion of responsibility for treatment success to the patient himself. This increasing patient involvement in the treatment process both depends upon and facilitates greater understanding on his part of psychosomatic events relevant to symptom development. ABT may also provide a useful tool for investigators exploring the interface between psychology and somatic medicine.

References

ACKNER, B.: The relationship between anxiety and the level of peripheral vasomotor activity. J. psychosom. Res. *1:* 21–48 (1956).

ADLER, C.S. and ADLER, S.M.: The pragmatic application of biofeedback to headaches. A five-year clinical follow-up. Proc. Biofeedback Research Society, p. 2 (University of Colorado Medical Center, Denver 1976).

ANTHONY, M. and LANCE, J.W.: Current concepts in the pathogenesis and interval treatment of migraine. Drugs *3:* 153–158 (1972).

APPENZELLER, O.: Vasomotor function in migraine. Headache *9:* 147–155 (1969).

BARLOW, D.H. and HERSEN, M.: Single case experimental designs. Uses in applied clinical research. Archs gen. Psychiat. *29:* 319–325 (1973).

BOUDEWYNS, P.A.: A comparison of the effects of stress versus relaxation instruction on the finger temperature response. Behav. Ther. *7:* 54–67 (1976).

BUDZYNSKI, T.; STOYVA, J. and ADLER, C.: Feedback-induced muscle relaxation. Application to tension headaches. J. Behav. Ther. exp. Psychiat. *1:* 205–211 (1970).

BURCH, G.E.; COHN, A.E. and NEUMAN, C.: A study by quantitative methods of the spontaneous variations in volume of the finger tip, toe tip, and posterior-superior portion of the pinna of resting normal white adults. Am. J. Physiol. *136:* 433–447 (1942).

DALESSIO, D.J.: Recent experimental studies on headache. Neurology *13:* 7–10 (1963).

DIAMOND, S. and FRANKLIN, M.: Biofeedback treatment choice in childhood migraine. Proc. Biofeedback Research Society, p. 13 (University of Colorado Medical Center, Denver 1976).

DICARA, L.V. and STONE, E.A.: The effect of instrumental heart-rate training on rat cardiac and brain catecholamines. Psychosom. Med. *32:* 359–368 (1970).

DRURY, R.L.; DERISI, W. and LIBERMAN, R.: Temperature feedback treatment for migraine headache. A controlled study. Proc. 5th Annual Biofeedback Research Society, p. 29 (University of Colorado Medical Center, Denver 1975).

ENGEL, R. and SCHAEFER, S.: Operant control of forehead skin temperature. Proc. 5th Annual Biofeedback Society, p. 38 (University of Colorado Medical Center, Denver 1974).

FIGAR, S.: Conditioned circulatory responses in men and animals; in Dow and HAMILTON Handbook of physiology, vol. 3, pp. 1991–2035 (Williams & Wilkins, Baltimore 1965).

Fowler, R.L. and Kimmel, H.D.: Operant conditioning of the GSR. J. exp. Psychol. 63: 563–567 (1962).

Friedman, A.P.: Reflection on the problem of headache. J. Am. med. Ass. 190: 445–447 (1964).

Graham, J.R. and Wolff, H.G.: Mechanism of migraine headache and action of ergotamine tartrate. Archs Neurol. Psychiat. 39: 737–763 (1938).

Green, E.E.; Green, A.M.; Walters, E.D.; Sargent, J.D., and Meyer, R.G.: Autogenic feedback training. Psychother. Psychosom. 25: 88–98 (1975).

Kazdin, A.E.: Methodological and assessment consideration in evaluating reinforcement programs in applied settings. J. Appl. Behav. Analysis 6: 517–531 (1973).

Koppman, J.W.; McDonald, R.D., and Kunzel, M.G.: Voluntary regulation of temporal artery diameter by migraine patients. Headache 14: 133–138 (1974).

Lacey, J.I. and Lacey, B.C.: The relationships of resting autonomic activity to motor impulsivity. The brain and human behavior (Williams & Wilkins, Baltimore 1958).

Leeb, C.; Fahrion, S. and French, D.: Instructional set, deep relaxation and growth enhancement. A pilot study. J. Humanist. Psychol. 16: 71–78 (1976).

Martin, M.J.; Rome, H.P. and Swenson, W.M.: Muscle-contraction headache. A psychiatric review, vol. 1, pp. 184–204 (Karger, Basel 1967).

Miller, N.E.: Learning of visceral and glandular responses. Science 163: 434–445 (1969).

Mittlemann, B. and Wolff, H.G.: Affective states and skin temperature. Experimental study of subjects with 'cold hands' and Raynaud's syndrome. Psychosom. Med. 1: 271–292 (1939).

Pearse, B.A.; Walter, E.D.; Sargent, J.D. and Meers, M.: Exploratory observations of the use of an intensive autogenic biofeedback training (IAFT) procedure in a follow-up study of out-of-town patients having migraine and/or tension headaches (Migraine Headache Project, Menninger Found., Topeka 1974).

Peper, E. and Grossman, E.R.: Preliminary observation of thermal biofeedback training in children with migraine. Proc. 5th Annual Biofeedback Research Society, p. 63 (University of Colorado Medical Center, Denver 1974).

Price, K.P. and Turskey, B.: Vascular reactivity in migraineurs and non-migraineurs. A comparison of responses to self-control procedures. Headache 16: 210–217 (1976).

Sargent, J.D.: Use of biofeedback in treatment of headache problems. Presented to the Texas Medical Association (Migraine Headache Project, Menninger Found., Topeka 1975).

Sargent, J.D.; Green, E.E. and Walters, E.D.: The use of autogenic feedback training in a pilot study of migraine and tension headaches. Headache 12: 120–124 (1972).

Sargent, J.D.; Walters, E.D., and Green, E.E.: Psychosomatic self-regulation of migraine headaches. Sem. Psychiat. 5: 415–428 (1973).

Savill, G.E. and Koppman, J.W.: Voluntary temporal artery regulation compared with finger blood volume and temperature. Proc. 6th Annual Biofeedback Research Society, p. 55 (University of Colorado Medical Center, Denver 1975).

Schultz, J.H. and Luthe, W.: Autogenic therapy, vol. 1 (Grune & Stratton, New York 1969).

Schumacher, G.A. and Wolff, H.G.: Experimental studies in headache. Archs Neurol. Psychiat. 45: 199–214 (1941).

Sicuteri, F.: Dry and wet theory in headache, vol. 3, pp. 159–165 (Karger, Basel 1972).

STERN, J.A.: Stability-lability of physiological response systems. Ann. N.Y. Acad. Sci. *134:* 1018–1027 (1966).
TAUB, E. and EMURIAN, C.S.: Feedback aided self-regulation of skin temperature with a single feedback locus. I. Acquisition and reversal training. Biofeedback Self-Regul. *1:* 147–168 (1976).
TURIN, A. and JOHNSON, W.G.: Biofeedback therapy for migraine headaches. Archs gen. Psychiat. *33:* 517–519 (1976).
WATERS, W.E. and O'CONNOR, P.J.: Prevalence of migraine. J. Neurol. Neurosurg. Psychiat. *38:* 613–616 (1975).
WICKRAMASKERA, I.E.: Temperature feedback for the control of migraine. J. Behav. Ther. exp. Psychiat. *4:* 343–345 (1973).
WOLFF, H.G.: Headache and other head pain; 2nd ed. (Oxford University Press, New York 1963).
ZAMANI, R.: Treatment of migraine headache. Biofeedback versus deep muscle relaxation. Research Report PR–785–2, Department of Psychiatry, Medical School (University of Minnesota, Minneapolis 1975).

STEVEN L. FAHRION, Ph.D., Department of Psychology, Mayo Clinic, *Rochester, MN 55901* (USA)

Acupuncture in Headache

J. J. Bischko[1]

Ludwig Boltzmann Acupuncture Institute, Vienna

All experienced acupuncturists report that it is possible to divide their cases into three, approximately equal groups: one third, headaches; one third, disorders of the locomotive apparatus; and one third, all those other medical conditions which can be treated by acupuncture. My own experience of 25 years, 19 of which have been devoted exclusively to acupuncture in a private practice and an outpatient clinic, confirms this distribution pattern.

Since 1973, over 3,000 new patients a year have attended the outpatient clinic of the Ludwig Boltzmann Acupuncture Institute. In that time we have seen 3,500 headache cases, but if private patients and those seen in earlier outpatient clinics are added, the total reaches 10,000.

I am unable to present exact statistics for the total case material because of the problems attending reexamination and follow-up. Many patients do not make the effort. Others, especially in private practice, are concerned about the costs of return visits (although, in fact, they are not charged). Despite this, one continues to hear, both directly and indirectly, frequent reports about the status of former patients. Most of these reports are positive but not infrequently they are negative.

In this report I will present the significant parameters derived from our experience. It is based on over 10% of the 10,000 headache cases treated. As headache in general, and migraine in particular, show such a wide spectrum of clinical pictures, I believe that any report dealing with less than 500 cases is relatively worthless.

Hopefully this report will be accepted not only for its scientific value but will stimulate others to critically pursue the use of acupuncture in headache.

[1] Diana-Reese-Soltész, Ludwig Boltzmann Acupuncture Institute, Vienna, assisted in the translation.

It might be expected that massive, detailed meaningful statistics on acupuncture would be available from China. Such is not the case. This is most unfortunate for acupuncture has been used there for several thousand years.

The history of European acupuncture starts in the 17th century with reports by the Dutch physician, TEN RHYNE [FEUCHT, 1976]. Later, acupuncture appears to have spread to other European countries with some concentration in France. Two interesting doctoral theses exist in the archives of the University of Vienna [FEUCHT, 1976]. One of these even discusses the use of electric current on the acupuncture points, utilizing Leyden jars for a power source. The patients' reactions were usually flight – some even jumped out of windows. FEUCHT is an excellent source of information on the history of acupuncture in Europe.

Acupuncture in the United States has, in contrast, a much shorter history. Following the initiation of political contact with the People's Republic of China by the NIXON administration, sensational reports on acupuncture began to appear in the American lay press. These prompted MILO D. LEAVITT, jr., MD, Director of the Fogarty International Center, Department of Health, Education and Welfare, National Institutes of Health, to invite three leading European acupuncturists to Bethesda, Maryland in December 1971 to review the state of the art. The experts were Dr. J.C. DE TYMOWSKI of Paris, France, at that time president of the 'Société Internationale d'Acupuncture', Dr. F. MANN of England and the author. Up to that time public discussion in the United States had concentrated on acupuncture analgesia, though a few immigrant MDs and Asiatic non-MDs were, in fact, actively practicing acupuncture therapy.

Because these first reports had dealt only with acupuncture analgesia, the impression at all scientific levels in the United States was that acupuncture was only a method for eliminating or reducing pain. As a consequence, the three European experts mentioned above had the distinct impression that they were considered during their American visit to be at best eccentrics and at worst crazy.

Almost complete confusion on the two major and distinct uses for acupuncture – analgesia and therapy – exists to this day in the United States.

The situation was further confused by publicity surrounding the inability of ROSEN [1974] to confirm Chinese claims for the effectiveness of acupuncture therapy for deaf and deaf-mute patients. These were the first reports to reach the United States on acupuncture therapy.

While we agree with ROSEN's findings with regard to objective criteria such as pre- and posttreatment audiograms, our own studies indicated that there were subjective parameters which had to be taken into account and which the Chinese had emphasized as being of significance.

In our studies, although the audiograms remained the same from pre- to posttreatment, the majority of cases showed subjectively better use of their remaining hearing capacity. (The only major exception was one patient in whom a 30% improvement was demonstrated on audiography.) Patients with no remnants of hearing capacity failed to show either objective or subjective change in our studies. ROSEN of course is also correct in emphasizing that the concepts of hard of hearing, deafness and even deaf-mutism can differ significantly in the People's Republic of China from what is acceptable in Western countries. Thus, KÖNIG [personal commun.] claims that about 80% of the children attending the Peking school for deaf-mutes would be able to attend normal schools in the West, where they would be fitted with hearing aids and accorded special treatment. Not being an otorhinolaryngologist I simply report this matter.

It is vital that the many differences between acupuncture for therapy and acupuncture for analgesia be recognized and understood. The major differences are indicated in table I.

While the differentiation shown in table I might be argued to be only indirectly related to the problem of headache, it is necessary to review this comparison between the methods and effects of acupuncture used for therapy and for analgesia before developing two basic statements:

(1) Headache should not be treated merely as a symptom. By using suitable acupuncture analgesia it is possible to achieve rapid sympathetic relief but not lasting improvement or healing. In such an application one is simply replacing the usually prescribed headache medication with needles.

(2) Seek the disorder which is causing headache, remembering that that disorder may not appear for some time after the manifestation of headache.

In the Chinese acupuncture literature – ancient and modern – pulse diagnosis is always employed as the principal and even the only method of determining the basic disorders. It takes at least 2 years for the average Western physician to become thoroughly familiar with pulse diagnosis. Despite recently developed electrical devices, the diagnostic value of pulse diagnosis is limited, approaching the 50% level in large measure because one third of all cases must be excluded on account of advanced arteriosclerosis, scars or deviations in the position of the normal pulse point of the radial artery.

The so-called Vienna School of Acupuncture recommends the use of

Table I. Differences between acupuncture therapy and acupuncture analgesia

Acupuncture therapy	Acupuncture analgesia
Point selection: very similar or the same Greater (up to 16) number of specific points	however, smaller number of specific loci smaller (up to 10)
Combination with auricular therapy is possible in both methods	however, more frequent in acupuncture analgesia
Needles are simply inserted and remain in place for 10–20 min; very rarely (except for paralyses) manual, vibratory, or electrical stimulation	continuous manual, vibratory, or electrical stimulation of the needles, otherwise, no effect produced (the technical parameters may be considered as known [BENZER et al., 1976]
Effect is general	effect is strictly local and limited in time (the extent to which dermatomes, myotomes, etc., play a role is the subject of continuing investigations)
Effect long-lasting, usually days or weeks, often months or years	effect short-lasting, hours at the most; limited after stimulation has been discontinued
Therefore, here the effect is not only neural, but without doubt, also humoral [RIEDERER et al., 1975]	effect is mainly neural; much literature exists on this subject [BENZER et al., 1976]
If electrical stimulation is used at all, then low voltage (up to 10–15 V) and low frequency (5–10 Hz) are used	particularly in combination analgesia with intubation and artificial immobilization, very high voltage (70 V and higher) as well as very different hertz values are employed
No significant additional medication	transition to electro-analgesia is not yet conclusively determined
Acupuncture alone under the above conditions produces a positive, lasting effect in the majority of cases, depending on the basic illness General use possible	only acupuncture combined with medication produces distinct effects (especially in major surgery); in minor surgery, acupuncture alone is sufficient general use not always possible (e.g. fearful patients or patients who do not react to acupuncture)
Effect lasts much longer Therefore, main method for headache	much shorter length of effect therefore, secondary method

pulse diagnosis (except in complicated cases [BISCHKO 1976]) as an adjunct to the taking of a thorough history and physical examination. It is essential that this detailed history include special consideration of certain modalities (to be discussed later) which are of importance in acupuncture. The taking of such a history is of course possible without any knowledge of pulse diagnosis.

Prof. DITTMAR of Badenweiler, West Germany, using patients with heart attacks as a model, claims that any pain leads to changes in catecholamines. Thus, acupuncture, which is painful even if only slightly so, could reduce the severity of a subsequent severe pain (as for example in a heart attack). Studies in which serotonin level changes were measured following acupuncture at various points, seem to confirm DITTMAR's assumption [1976] and underline the work of KELLNER [1966].

At the Institute a long-term series of studies have been underway on the effects of acupuncture on catecholamines. Some of these studies seem to contradict the work of DITTMAR.

Under normal acupuncture conditions a red ring appears in the skin around the needle after insertion. The red ring develops different sizes and color intensity while the needle stays in the tissues. The smaller the diameter of the needle (as for example with thin high quality steel) the less marked the reaction. The greater the diameter (as is seen with those needles made of precious metals such as gold and/or silver) the greater the reaction. In addition, the reaction tends to be greater when acupuncture is performed on skin that is usually covered (e.g., abdomen, inner side of the upper arm or thighs) than when it is conducted on skin that is normally exposed (e.g., lower legs, lower arms or hands, face).

In one recent experiment we took a group of patients of both sexes (age range 26–63) and pretreated them with large parenteral doses of antihistamines. In addition, shortly before insertion of the needles, we applied antihistamine salves to the points to be acupunctured. Despite the relatively high parenteral and local application of antihistamines the red rings appeared and were only reduced in size and color intensity by less than 10% compared with normals. Two separate teams at the Institute are currently using techniques employing cannulas which remain *in situ* while a double-blind study is conducted of blood histamine levels before, during and after acupuncture together with an evaluation of placebo effects.

We believe (see table I) that much greater significance can be attached to the biochemical findings in acupuncture therapy than in acupuncture analgesia where the effects are more related to the neural stimulation. In therapy there is an initial neural impact but the ultimate effects are far more broad and general. Indeed, if the peripheral nervous system is completely destroyed or temporarily blocked by any mechanism such as drugs, acupuncture is totally or almost completely ineffective. In transsection of the cord, for example, while acupuncture is able to produce changes which are perceived as distinct, though slight alleviations by the patient, the relief is restricted to the specific segment or dermatome acupunctured. We have found that the effect of the acupuncture in such a case is transmitted neither cranially nor caudally.

There is an old German saying: 'Every theory is grey, but the tree of life is green.' Let us turn then from theories and research to our 'tree of life', the practice of acupuncture.

Although acupuncture originated in China, Western physicians should not slavishly accept as superior everything emanating from there or especially from Taiwan, Hong Kong, Japan or other Far Eastern countries. Although all these countries have had much longer experience with acupuncture, their practice has been tailored to Asiatics. Research, as we in the West understand it, is carried out to some extent in the People's Republic of China, less so in Japan and not at all elsewhere in the Far East.

There are several other reasons for the development of significant differences between the practice of acupuncture in the West and the Far East. Without research, medical methods are at best empirical. The level of education of the practitioner may dictate certain modifications. For example, because the so-called barefoot doctors (who are not of course doctors) possess only rudimentary medical knowledge, the Chinese in their text books have deliberately relocated many acupuncture points to avoid injuring vessels, pleura, peritoneum, articular capsules, etc. It may even be that the body structure of the Easterner, including for example the length and form of the intestinal tract, is different from that of Westerners.

Because of these differences, the Vienna School of Acupuncture has sought to develop a specific, Western, European form of acupuncture. To achieve this we explored pathophysiological laws in each particular type of case. While the details may seem a little boring it is necessary to review systematically and in detail the basis upon which the Vienna School has based its practice.

There must be as many classifications of headache as there are types of treatment. In treating headache by acupuncture we utilize a method of classification such as that developed by my colleague, Dr. M. KRÖTLINGER

[1976]. We believe that careful case history taking and examination are essential. We pay special attention to such matters as:

(1) The specific location of the pain or attack.

(2) Whether or not the pain is unilateral and whether or not there has been a history of some sort of alternation of sides with regard to the pain.

(3) Other modalities which we believe can produce or aggravate the severity of an attack such as menstruation, ovulation, weather influences, psychic alterations, to name but a few, together with more widely recognized influences such as nutrition, alcohol and/or drug use and abuse, excessive smoking, etc.

A basic knowledge of acupuncture and the location of its points is of course essential.

As a necessary precursor to identifying the correct acupuncture modality we classify the headache into one of four groups according to the site and spread of pain:

(1) A frontal group. Here we consider those headaches which start in the region of the eye (ophthalmic migraine is included) and either stay in the frontal region or radiate dorsally. There are two subgroups: (a) where the pain radiates over the top of the head to the occipital region (acupuncturists would describe this as following the Meridian of the Bladder), and (b) where it radiates laterally, moving temporally from the region of the eye to end behind the auricle.

(2) A temporoparietal group. In this group, the pain starts in the temple area and usually radiates behind the ear but in some cases may radiate towards the lateral angle of the orbit. In female patients with such a 'temporal' headache, one can almost always demonstrate a correlation with menstruation or ovulation and a negative correlation with pregnancy.

(3) A vertical group. The pain starts at or near the vertex of the skull and spreads downwards on all sides covering an area like a cap. All these cases we associate with intestinal disorders.

(4) A dorsal group where the pain begins either occipitally, nuchally or even cervically, before radiating anteriorly (usually over the vertex or only rarely temporally). In such cases treatment must also be aimed at the cervical (and often the cervicobrachial) region.

It must be stressed that there is only a slight difference in the specifics of acupuncture therapy for migraine and for other forms of headache. (This is comparable to the situation that exists where the treatment specifics for gastric and duodenal ulcer are almost identical).

The alternating appearance of pain in the left or right half of the head (as in migraine) is unimportant for acupuncture for the main points are always acupunctured bilaterally. When headache occurs predominantly on one side, extra individual points are acupunctured unilaterally on the ipsilateral side. The situation is different, however, in those rare cases of migraine where the headache invariably manifests itself on one side. In such cases a single needle is used (Lu 7)[2] as a main point on the contralateral side.

Much emphasis is placed on other modalities which comprise a larger diagnostic group: this is the group of headaches which is dependent upon other factors such as the environment. Acupuncturists believe that all illnesses – in the case of the present paper, all headaches – can be triggered or aggravated by exogenous or endogenous factors.

The influences of these various exogenous or endogenous factors dictate the specific sites at which one elects to conduct acupuncture intervention.

(1) In headaches dependent upon female hormonal influences (mentioned earlier) we know that points 3H 22 (also termed G-3 as intersection point) as well as PV 16 and B 31 are effective for therapy. Indeed, acupuncture at point 3H 22 appears to work by delaying significantly the onset of menstruation itself.

(2) The weather, or more specifically changes in the weather, plays a role in causing headache. Many patients can anticipate changes even 24–48 h (and rarely up to 76 h) before the actual weather changes. Although general practitioners in many countries claim to have seen weather-related phenomena, such as an increase in heart attacks, thrombosis, etc., there has apparently been little research and less in the way of publications on this fascinating topic.

The work of MARESCH [1966] is interesting in this regard. It is based on the observation that patients perceive changes in weather less through barometric changes than through a combination of a jump in humidity and inversion. (Inversion means the change or even reversal of the old physical law that temperature drops about 5.5°C for every 1 km altitude increase.)

According to MARESCH the simultaneous occurrence of an increase in humidity and of inversion leads to a change in the electric field of the earth, which normally totals about 150 V/1 m altitude. (Another incidental result

---

[2] Obviously, an important aspect of acupuncture is the identification of the specific acupuncture sites. Rather than include all details in the text, all sites referred to are listed in an 'Appendix' in the order in which they appear in the text.

of such a dual occurrence is the reduction of emission of dust, soot and other particles.) A person of normal height moves about in an electric field which roughly corresponds with the intensity of the usual commercial current (in Europe) of 220 V. As acupuncture points show reduced skin resistance (which is why they are called 'electrically superior points of the skin'), they can be considered more or less as entrance gates for any field charge which occurs with drastic weather changes.

(3) Psychological factors are widely recognized as playing a role in the genesis or aggravation of headache, especially migraine. It is widely believed that such clinical manipulation must be radiated through some chemical substances such as histamine or serotonin. Acupuncturists believe that acupuncture therapy must be a/the regulative therapy in physiological and pathophysiological terms.

(4) As mentioned earlier, conditions of misuse or abuse of alcohol, nicotine or other drugs must also be taken into account, as must faulty nutrition.

The reader will be interested in finding out how to use acupuncture within the conditions mentioned above, which points should be selected, and how they should be combined or varied. It must be stressed that any 'collection of recipes' ignores the essence of acupuncture, for despite the fact that congruous parameters exist, there is no absolute individuality.

Before outlining certain standard combinations it is necessary to emphasize some basic facts. Every point has the capacity for impact in several ways or rather at several levels:

(1) Local means that it acts on the area of the body under which the point lies.

(2) Regional applies to action on a dermatome, extremity, etc.

(3) Superregional: this refers to an action which may be perceptible far beyond the region of the point. While this is clinically proven, the biochemical or neurophysiological mechanisms of action have yet to be demonstrated.

(4) There are, in addition, some acupuncture points which traditionally have been known to have a generalized effect. Such points occupy actual finite areas rather than specific, localized spots and one can often demonstrate so-called satellite points. In China these are often called new and extra points. We have shown that these 'new' points have such a close relationship to well-known, long established 'general' points, as far as location and indications are concerned, that today we should only speak of satellite points.

PETRICEK and ZEITLER [1976] have developed a new computer-oriented nomenclature for them. Thus, if a point lies approximately in the region of

St 36 on the Meridian of the Stomach, we call the point on the meridian lying closest to it, St 36-1. However, if the point lying closest to St 36 lies lateral or medial to it we call it St 36-01. This new nomenclature, which takes into consideration later computer analysis, not only simply replaces such complicated terms as 'new point' or 'extra point' but also makes it easier for a student to deal with the subject.

After this major preamble it is appropriate to list the most important points and their common combinations:

(1) The main points for frontal migraine are: SI 4, St 36, St 41, possibly St 44, B 1, B 2, PdM, G 3, G 14. If this basic combination does not produce the desired effect within a reasonable amount of time, one can add the following points individually or combined: B 60, B 10, G 20, PV 19, PV 23.

(2) The main points for temporoparietal migraine are: G 3, G 17, G 40, G 43, B 2, B 64, B 67. Additional points are: B 60, B 10, G 20, PV 19, PV 23.

(3) The main points for cervical migraine are: B 1, B 2, B 4, B 10, G 20, PV 13, PV 19. Additional points are: B 60, LI 4, SI 3, 3H 15.

(4) The main points for other headaches are: PV 19, PV 23, B 1, B 2, B 10, G 3, G 20. Additional points are: B 60, LI 4, SI 3, Lu 7.

The above point combinations are those that we have found to be most effective for all cases of the same type. However, where individuals have special problems or one or more of the four special factors discussed earlier are predominant, it may be necessary to use alternative acupuncture points.

It is possible to tackle the special factors as follows:

(1) Hormonal influences. The points PV 16, B 31, K 11, PV 4, and 3H 22 are used most often, either alone or in combination. No more than 16 needles (i.e. the use of 8–11 different points) should be used at one time during one session. The less needles per treatment, carefully selected, the greater the effect.

(2) Weather changes. One significant point 3H 15 changes sensibility to weather.

(3) Psychological influences. The points CV 15, PV 19 and PV 20 are recommended as the basic treatment for psychic parameters. Where vegetative dystonia dominates, points B 10 and G 20 are used simultaneously. For primary or secondary depression, points H 3 and CV 6 are useful and less frequently B 39.

(4) The treatment of nutritional errors, alcohol, nicotine or drug abuse requires greater variations and demands more experience. In these cases auricular therapy with the aggression points, the lung and stomach zones can often be effective.

It would be beyond the scope of this article to list all possible point combinations for the disorders discussed. It is most unfortunate that there are no books in English based on a modern pathophysiological approach to acupuncture. Those books presently available are based either on ancient texts (e.g. Nei-Ching and Su-Wenn) or modern reflexology which cannot always be carried out in Western countries for legal reasons (e.g. pinching the axillary nerve in cases of frozen shoulder).

In the absence of such texts, it is valuable to consider the many points on a basis of functional groups. For all headaches it is possible to consider the points roughly according to their primary action in:

(1) Improving the blood supply of the head.

(2) Harmonizing the production of hormones.

(3) Changing faulty flow relationship in the vascular supply of the head.

(4) Delving into specific psychological parameters (e.g. nightmares via St 44 etc.).

(5) Developing psychological balance.

(6) The so-called personal points, which are seen especially in cervical migraine are points identified by the patient. They can lie on or outside the meridian and should always be included in a treatment session if the patient indicates their existence. As they are usually no longer evident by the following session, there is a parallel to auricular therapy.

Of course, any one point can be effective as part of two or more functional groups. As a consequence, one is well-advised to select points which act on as many groups as possible. This, of course, keeps down the total number of needles used at any one time.

Conclusion

Even apart from its specific effectiveness in the treatment of headaches (including migraine) the wide spectrum of acupuncture can greatly aid the therapist faced with the wide variety of disorders or factors which produce headache as a symptom. The acupuncturist is required to have considerable special knowledge, such as the mechanism of action of the various points. We believe that the synthesis of the Vienna School of Acupuncture can greatly aid the orthodox, causally trained Western physician to become familiar and achieve therapeutic success with acupuncture. Scientific research especially on pain is now being carried out all over the world.

References

Benzer, H.; Bischko, J.; Pauser, G. und Zimmermann, M.: Die Akupunktur-Analgesie; in Benzer, Frey, Hügin und Mayrhofer Lehrbuch der Anästhesiologie, Reanimation und Intensivtherapie, pp. 403–409 (Springer, Berlin 1976).

Bischko, J.: Einführung in die Akupunktur; 8th ed. (Haug, Heidelberg 1976a).

Bischko, J.: Akupunktur für Fortgeschrittene; 5th ed. (Haug, Heidelberg 1976b).

Bischko, J.: Akupunktur für mässig Fortgeschrittene (Haug, Heidelberg, in press).

Dittmar, F.: Zeitkrankheit Herzinfarkt. Ärztl. Prax. 28: 2397 (1976).

Feucht, G.: Geschichte der Akupunktur in Europa; in Bischko Handbuch der Akupunktur und Aurikulotherapie (Haug, Heidelberg 1976).

Kellner, G.: Bau und Funktion der Haut. Dt. Z. Akupunktur 15: 1–31 (1966).

Krötlinger, M.: Akupunktur in der Allgemeinpraxis; in Bischko Handbuch der Akupunktur und Aurikulotherapie (Haug, Heidelberg 1976).

Maresch, O.: Das Elektrische Verhalten der Haut. Dt. Z. Akupunktur 15: 33–50 (1966).

Petricek, E. und Zeitler, H.: Neue systematische Ordnung der Neu-Punkte; in Bischko Handbuch der Akupunktur und Aurikulotherapie (Haug, Heidelberg 1976).

Riederer, P.; Tenk, H.; Werner, H.; Bischko, J.; Rett, A., and Krisper, H.: Manipulation of neurotransmitters by acupuncture. A preliminary communication. J. neural Transmis. 37: 81–94 (1975).

Rosen, S.: Feasibility of acupuncture as a treatment for sensori-neural deafness in children. Laryngoscope 84: 2202–2217 (1974).

Appendix

List of Points Mentioned in Text in the Order of Their First Appearance

Point	Location
Lu 7 (Lung 7)	in the radial indentation, just a crossfinger proximal to the capitulum radii, that is, somewhat above the 3rd pulse position
3H 22 [Triple Heater (Warmer) 22]	half a crossfinger above the middle of the os zygomaticum
G 3 (Gallbladder 3)	see 3H 22
PV 16 (Pilot Vessel 16)	on the median line, on the lower edge of the occiput
B 31 (Bladder 31)	in the first sacral foramen in its distal, medial quadrant
St 36 (Stomach 36)	on the point of intersection of the lines half a crossfinger lateral to the linea interossea of the tibia, and 2 crossfingers below the head of the fibula, that is, between m. tibialis anterior and m. extensor digit. longus
SI 4 (Small Intestine 4)	on the lateral edge of the hand over the articular space of the 5th metacarpal bone and the os hamatum
St 41 (Stomach 41)	on the lower edge of the tiba, in the middle of the tarsus
St 44 (Stomach 44)	proximal to the angle of the base joint of the 2nd and 3rd toes
B 1 (Bladder 1)	in the angle formed by the root of the nose and the orbit
B 2 (Bladder 2)	on the foramina supraorbitalis
B 64 (Bladder 64)	on the outer edge of the foot, immediately proximal to the base joint of the 5th toe
B 67 (Bladder 67)	2 mm proximal and lateral to the outer angle of the toenail of the small toe; acupuncture of this point is quite painful
B 4 (Bladder 4)	somewhat more than 2 crossfingers above the hairline (or where it used to be, which can usually be determined by the different skin color)
PV 13 (Pilot Vessel 13)	on the 7th cervical vertebra
LI 4 (Large Instestine 4)	in the proximal angle between the 1st and 2nd metacarpal bones on the dorsum manus
SI 3 (Small Intestine 3)	when the hand is closed in a fist, this point lies on the lateral end of the skin fold which is formed behind (proximal to) the base joint of the small finger
3 H 15 [Triple Heater (Warmer) 15]	this point usually lies on the upper trapezial edge in the middle of the shoulder, however, it can sometimes lie 1–2 crossfingers deeper and somewhat lateral to this location; it is so sensitive to pressure, especially in persons who are sensitive to weather, that locating it presents no difficulty
K 11 (Kidney 11)	on the upper edge of the pubis, 2 crossfingers lateral to the symphysis
PV 4 (Pilot Vessel 4)	on the 3rd lumbar vertebra, thus, relatively deep if one exactly observes the spinal process

Point	Location
PdM (Point de merveille)	in the middle of the root of the nose
G 14 (Gallbladder 14)	the intersection of an imaginary vertical line through the pupil of the eye and a line 2 crossfingers above the eyebrow
B 60 (Bladder 60)	on the upper, lateral edge of the calcaneum in the middle of an imaginary line between the malleolus externus and the Achilles tendon
B 10 (Bladder 10)	on the lower edge of the occiput, 2 crossfingers outside the dorsal median line; at this same distance, all the following points up to B 27 are found
G 20 (Gallbladder 20)	on the lower occipital edge, just behind the mastoid
PV 19 (Pilot Vessel 19)	in the median line on the point of intersection of the lambda and sagittal sutures in the indentation; warning: do not insert the needle too far into this point!
PV 23 (Pilot Vessel 23)	in the middle of the root of the nose on the point of intersection with the eyebrows
G 17 (Gallbladder 17)	3 crossfingers lateral to the point of intersection of a horizontal line through the uppermost tip of the pinna and the median line over the skull
G 40 (Gallbladder 40)	difficult to find, over the calcaneocuboid joint
G 43 (Gallbladder 43)	on the lateral side of the base joint of the 4th toe, over the articular space
CV 15 (Conc. Vessel 15)	immediately below the tip of the xiphoid
PV 20 (Pilot Vessel 20)	on the median line, on the uppermost point of the crown of the head
H 3 (Heart 3)	when the arm is maximally bent, we find this point on the medial end of the crease of the elbow; it is easy to find and frequently used
CV 6 (Conc. Vessel 6)	in the middle of the fourth fifth above the symphysis (of the distance between symphysis and navel); on thin persons 2 crossfingers below the navel
B 39 (Bladder 39)	locating this point is somewhat complicated; the easiest method is to have the patient sit with legs and knees close together, resting his elbows on his knees, thus forming an arched back; now the point, on the point of intersection of the scapula and the upper edge of the 4th rib is accessible; in a normal posture, it is covered by the scapula

Dr. JOHANNES BISCHKO, L. Boltzmann-Institut für Akupunktur, Allgemeine Poliklinik, Mariannengasse 10, *A–1090 Wien* (Austria)

Cryosurgery of Headache

NORMAN COOK

Royal Jubilee Hospital, Victoria, B.C.

Contents

Introduction 86
Development of Procedure 87
Rationale 87
Indications 88
Contraindications 88
Results 88
Anatomic and other Considerations 90
Surgery 91
Phenomena Observed during Cryosurgery in the Sphenopalatine Area 94
Animal Experiments... 96
The Transantral Approach 99
Complications 99
Postoperative Course 100
Summary 101
References 101

Introduction

Many attacks of headache, whether they be classified as migraine or cluster headache, will feature pain in or around the orbit, mainly behind the eye. This pain usually can be quickly relieved by the application of a local anesthetic such as cocaine on a cotton-tipped flexible applicator high in the back of the nose over the sphenopalatine area. If the pain is accompanied by a wet eye and ptosis, these will usually disappear also.

To find a method whereby this transient relief might be prolonged to a practical degree has challenged researchers, including myself, for many years. This search has led to the use of cryosurgery in the treatment of headache.

GREENFIELD SLUDER [1] was probably the first to focus attention upon the sphenopalatine autonomic complex in relation to headache and he coined the term 'nasal ganglion neuralgia'. His description of the headache suggests that many of his cases were cluster headache as we now know this condition. If he was able to stop the patient's acute attack with cocaine in the back of the nose he would then proceed to inject the area of the sphenopalatine ganglion with a mixture of phenol and alcohol. His use of this procedure met with a measure of success but it has been discarded as a practical treatment in this type of headache.

Development of Procedure

Cryosurgery has been used by this author for some time in cases of intractable Ménière's disease using the method originally described by WOLFSON *et al.* [2]. This consists of freezing the thinned out horizontal semicircular canal and producing a selective labyrinthectomy.

Encouraged by the results in Ménière's disease, the same small 2.75 mm cryoprobe was used by myself in 1968 with some cautious timidity in the region of the sphenopalatine (SP) foramen in a case of cluster headache which had been *unremitting*. When this patient, several months later, reported relief from pain I was encouraged to use the procedure in other cases of headache. It is the purpose of this article to report the observations and results of the use of cryosurgery in various kinds of headache (approximately 684 procedures) during the last 8 years.

Rationale

Peripheral nerves are notoriously vulnerable to cryosurgery but recovery usually takes place sooner or later. It is my opinion that autonomic nerves are even more susceptible and that if the probe is accurately placed on target, recovery is much less likely to occur. A cryo-needle for the appeasement of peripheral nerve pain was reported by LLOYD *et al.* [3] in 1976. Vasomotor rhinitis (a common autonomic disorder within the nose) has responded very well to cryosurgery as pioneered by OZENBERGER [4]. I have found his method very satisfactory and it has been adopted by many other otolaryngologists.

It is possible that freezing branches of the external carotid artery is superior to cutting these arteries because the freezing effect extends outside the artery wall and seems to have a lethal effect on the autonomic nerve accompaniment of the artery. I personally suspect that the procedure produces a 'peripheral sympathectomy'.

Indications

An ideal case might be:
(1) Typical unilateral severe migraine in a reasonably stable person.
(2) Cluster headache which is inadequately controlled by drugs. (One should beware of a definitely hostile personality.)

Contraindications

(1) Bilateral migrainous headache.
(2) 'Ping-pong' headache in which migraine attacks alternate from side to side.
(3) Typical migraine which starts on one side and then transfers itself to the other side for the rest of the attack.
(4) Menstrual migraine.
(5) Posttraumatic migrainous headache, which may resemble typical migraine except for the history of trauma prior to the onset of headaches.
(6) Psychogenic headache. Here, only an occasional satisfactory result has been achieved with cryosurgery. However, one cannot expect migraineurs to be other than volatile to some extent. It is a matter of judgement.
(7) If one suspects that the patient blames all his inadequacies on his headache, a good result is unlikely.
(8) Recurring serious depression.

Results

At the end of 8 months, all patients receive a follow-up questionnaire which is worded as follows: (1) Do you consider the result of your operation 8 months ago to be a failure? (2) If on the successful side, would you estimate your improvement to be 25, 50, 75 or 100%? (3) Additional remarks.

554 patients gave definite answers to the above questions. The results are as follows: failure, 180; improvement, 25% = 29; 50% = 67; 75% = 116; 100% = 162.

The remaining 130 cases involved mostly repeat operations and a few who answered the questionnaire in so much detail that I could not assess their result.

With a highly diluted diagnosis one must allow for the power of suggestion and for recurrence after the patient has returned the follow-up questionnaire. Undoubtedly, many of the patients with good results have subsequently had a recurrence of headache. A few of the patients with poor results (25% or less improvement) later reported a good result.

Although the results are obviously not mathematically accurate, I can summarize the results with what I consider to be a conservative statement, that a definite *majority* have achieved a practical improvement.

The recurrence rate in cluster headache is higher than in common migraine. When a cluster headache patient is free of headache for months after cryosurgery and then the headache recurs, one may wonder if the original surgical result may have been a natural remission. Due allowance has been made for this. It is gratifying to receive occasional reports from patients who have now been free of cluster headache (with previously little or no natural remissions) for as long as 6 years.

If cryosurgery seemed successful for a year or two, but failed to produce a lasting result, one may resort to the transantral procedure (which in a few cases has produced several headache free years); or one may apply cryosurgery to the sphenopalatine area in a gentle manner using a short freeze and a short reproduction when the cluster begins (this method has also met with sucess.) In such a case, the freezing is just sufficient to abort the cluster which the patient is entering.

Some of the cases which are contained in the above-mentioned results of cryosurgery do not belong in a diagnostic 'pigeon hole'. Many of these patients would probably be diagnosed as tension headache. I have paid much more attention to the location of the headache in terms of three branches of the external carotid artery, namely the sphenopalatine, the superficial temporal and the occipital which, in my opinion, are involved in most cases of hemicrania or cluster headache. If I were to confine the procedure to the ideal cases described in 'Indications', I think the results would be much better than the highly diluted group which I am recording here.

Anatomic and other Considerations

The external carotid artery ends by dividing into the superficial temporal and internal maxillary arteries. The terminal branch of the maxillary artery is the SP which enters the nose through the SP foramen and controls most of the ever changing blood supply to the nose. *This artery always lies in front of and in close proximity to the SP ganglion.* It is likely that the cryoprobe, if accurately placed, will freeze both artery and ganglion at the same time.

The SP ganglion has attracted surgical attention for years, but removal of the ganglion does not seem to have achieved the desired result.

Since the superficial temporal and occipital branches of the external carotid artery seem to contribute an important part to the pain in migraine, and even in cluster headache, and since there is no ganglion involved in either of these two arteries, one wonders if the SP *artery* may be the offender in some types of migraine and cluster headache which feature pain behind the eye. The artery may impart its disturbance to the ganglion with which it is in such intimate contact. Anyone who has observed the angry edema surrounding the superficial temporal artery during an attack of some types of headache can imagine the reaction which probably also surrounds the maxillary and SP artery.

The maxillary artery is mysteriously tortuous. Its branches close to the nose in the SP fossa are coiled together like a 'bag of worms' in proximity to the ganglion. I have removed a block of tissue from cadavers, including the 'bag of worms', and sections through this tissue show a great surfeit of nerve fibres which follow the twists and turns of these arteries. Presumably these are sympathetic fibres since they cling to and follow the course of the arteries. The complexity of this arterial and autonomic plexus may explain some of the surgical failures (including cryosurgery).

If one successfully freezes *only* the SP area, it is likely that the orbital (usually retrobulbar) pain will be relieved along with the wet eye and ptosis, but it is also likely that attacks of pain will continue in the distribution of the superficial temporal artery. Therefore, I always freeze them both at the same time and if the occipital branch seems to contribute to the clinical picture, all three are frozen at one operation which I have come to call the 'hemicrania' procedure, which has now become almost routine. Involvment of the occipital artery may show itself only as a tightening of the muscles at the back of the head, sometimes almost down to the shoulder.

In migraine, or occasionally in cluster headache, one of these three arteries may appear to be operating alone in causing symptoms. The pain and vasodilatation may seem to be due, for instance, entirely to the superficial temporal, but the results obtained by freezing the superficial temporal alone are usually disappointing except for a temporary improvement. While freezing, under local anesthetic, the SP area in the nose, the reproduction of pain is often at the front of the temple or at times in the occiput, and freezing in the occiput will occasionally produce a pain above or behind the eye. Thus, it seems that the carotid system behaves as a unit, with reciprocity between these branches and even across to the other side of the head. For instance, if a patient volunteers that a migraine attack involves the left side 80% of the time and the right side 20%, he should be warned that cryosurgery, if successful on the severely affected side, may seem to aggravate headache on the other side. Many of the repeat operations have been on the other side. Because of the reaction to the cryosurgical procedure, to be described later, it is not wise to do both sides of the head at once. As stated earlier in this report, the ideal case is unilateral.

SAXENA [5] in his outstanding research demonstrated in dogs the selective response of the carotid system, as compared to other arteries, to specific drugs such as ergotamine. He also found that cervical sympathectomy in these dogs definitely altered the response to ergotamine.

In the SP prodecedure, if the probe is close enough to the target area (artery and ganglion), the patient will experience a quick reproduction of his own pain behind or around the eye. Occasionally he may feel this pain in the temple or in the occiput, or if the tip of the probe is lowered by a millimeter or so, the pain may be felt in the maxilla. *This reproduction of the patient's pain is essential to a good result.* Sometimes, it is necessary to try various positions of the probe in order to obtain the desired reproduction of pain.

Local anesthetic is essential. It permits the patient and surgeon to be in communication with each other. If the pain is too severe, the temperature is raised or the nitrogen feed is cut off until the reproduced pain fades away. Then the freezing is repeated possibly four or five times until, finally, the patient can easily tolerate a 5-min freeze without too much pain.

Surgery

The following report describes a fairly typical cryosurgical procedure.

The pulse of the occipital artery on the left side was felt with the finger just below the occipital bone and just behind the mastoid bone in the soft notch between the sternomastoid and trapezius muscles. This was marked with a needle dipped in methylene blue. An incision of 0.5 cm was made and then spread with forceps down to fascia, but the vessel was not exposed. A 4.7-mm cryosurgical probe was pressed over the vessel and the temperature dropped to $-130°C$ and held for 3 min. A period of thaw was then allowed and the same freeze was repeated again.

A similar procedure was carried out over the left superficial temporal vessel above the zygoma. A temperature of $-120°C$ was used for 2 min followed by a thaw and a repeat freeze. Each incision was closed with a single buried catgut suture and a small bandaid was applied.

During the above procedure, the nose was under cocaine crystal anesthesia which was applied as follows:

Flexible wire applicators wound with cotton at the tips were dampened with epinephrine 1 in 1000 and then rolled in crystals (flakes) of cocaine. One of these was placed between the middle turbinate and the septum, over the SP area. Another was placed underneath the middle turbinate at the back of the middle meatus. A third was placed between the front of the middle turbinate and the septum to block the anterior ethmoidal nerves. The probe size was now changed to 3.2 mm. This probe has a slight curve. Underneath the middle turbinate at the back of the middle meatus a small nasal forceps was introduced to invade the posterior ethmoid close to the turbinate. The back of the tunnel would be the body of the sphenoid bone. Into this tunnel the small probe was placed and the temperature dropped to $-160°C$. Little or no reproduction of the patient's retrobulbar headache was obtained. Then a small tunnel was made through the middle turbinate near its posterior end into the substance of the turbinate and possibly some surface ethmoid cells. When the probe was placed in this tunnel at $-60°C$ an immediate reproduction of the patient's pain behind the eye was obtained. Because the pain was severe, the nitrogen feed was switched off at the end of about 1 min. The freeze was repeated four times with increasing tolerance to the pain and finally the last freeze lasted 5 min at $-160°C$ with only moderate reproduction of the pain behind the eye. This completed the operation.

Reference is made here to figure 1 which shows occipital and superficial temporal positions. Figure 2 shows three approaches to the SP area. The position on the far right is to be condemned because the probe here is not buried in insulating bone but is placed between middle turbinate and septum and though far behind the main olfactory area, it has destroyed the sense of smell. This position has been completely abandoned. Figure 3 shows

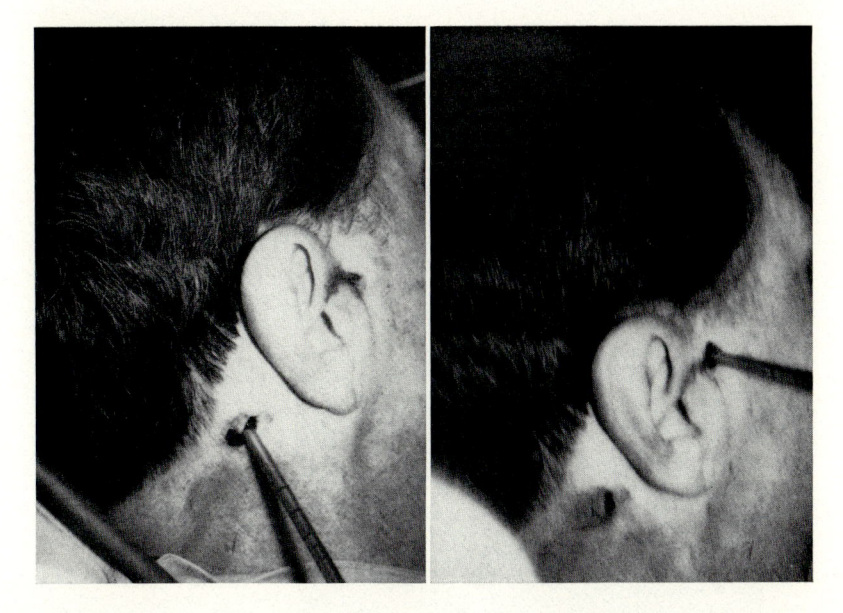

Fig. 1. Occipital and superficial temporal procedures. The occipital procedure has, in a few cases, caused a sudden dilatation of the pupil of the eye on that side.

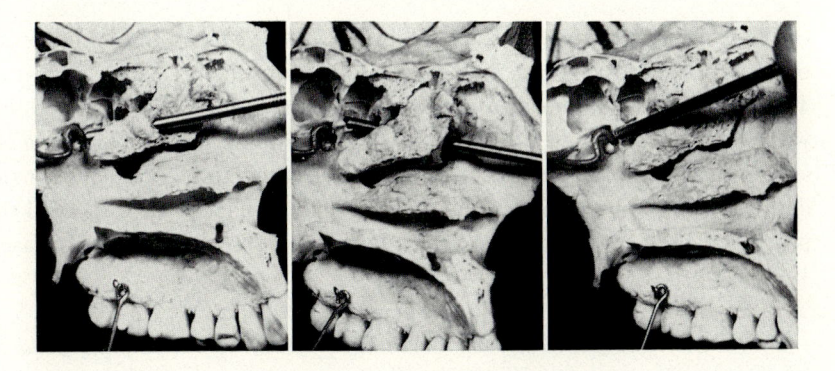

Fig. 2. On the far left, the probe is shown in the substance of the turbinate. In the center, the probe is shown in the ethmoid position. The position shown on the far right, in which the probe is not buried in any insulating bone, has been abandoned because of damage to the sense of smell.

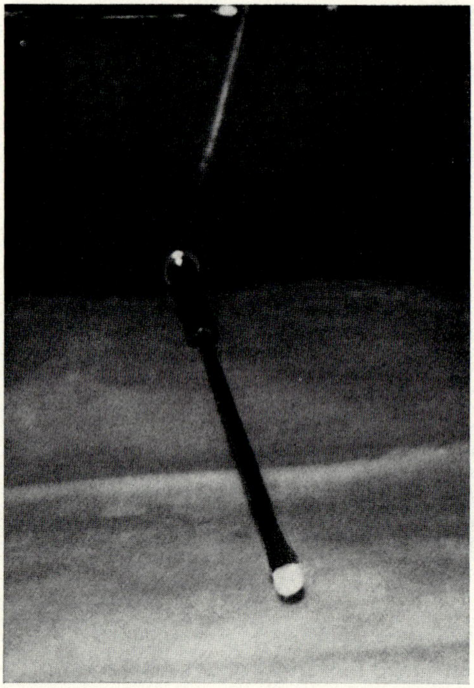

Fig. 3. Shows the large probe at –160°C activated. Note that freezing takes place at the tip. The shank of the probe is vacuum insulated.

the large 4.7-mm probe activated at –160°C. It will be seen that only the tip of the probe is freezing because the shank of the probe is vacuum insulated. The machine uses liquid nitrogen which boils at –196°C and it is possible with this machine to go as low as –190°C during the operation. In the SP area within the nose a temperature of –160°C seems to be optimum for the desired results to be achieved. Other otolaryngologists who have adopted the procedure have settled upon the same temperature in the majority of cases.

Phenomena Observed during Cryosurgery in the Sphenopalatine Area

In one case a mechanical dysfunction occurred and the temperature at the probe tip went below –190°C. This was about 6 years ago and at that time a large probe was being used in the nose. The patient's pain was immediately reproduced very severely and on the fourth freeze his pupil dilated to the fullest possible extent. Among the numerous names which are used for what we now call cluster headache, is the name 'ciliary neuralgia'. In this case, and in others undergoing cryosurgery in the SP area, a change in the size of the pupil suggests that, somehow or another, the cold impulse has managed to reach the ciliary ganglion. Postoperatively this patient developed a third nerve diplopia which lasted 3½ weeks and then cleared. His disabling retrobulbar headache has been relieved now for about 6 years.

During the SP freeze, providing the probe is close enough on target, one may expect a complete or partial reproduction of this syndrome, if any one of the following symptoms is a feature of each attack of headache: – (1) extreme nausea and vomiting; (2) paresthesiae, usually in the upper limb and amounting to a diagnosis of hemiplegic migraine; (3) scotomata, which may be colored or otherwise, appearing with headaches; (4) hallucinations occurring with each attack of headache, and (5) blurred vision or double vision with each attack of headache.

Figure 4 shows a chart of temperature and time drawn by the machine during cryosurgery for severe migraine in a patient whose attacks featured vomiting. The chart reads from below upward. The first two freezes at $-160°C$ were in the now forbidden position between the middle turbinate and the septum, a procedure which in some patients has destroyed the sense of smell. Such was the case in this patient. The reproduction of her pain in this position was poor. Then the probe was moved into the ethmoid and a reproduction of her pain was instantly obtained as well as immediate nausea which amounted to vomiting and forced me to stop the freeze two or three times. Before the last freeze, a Stellate ganglion block was performed by one of the anesthetists producing a Horner's syndrome and a difference in temperature between the two hands. It was then possible for me to freeze at $-160°C$ for as long as I wished, with no nausea appearing at all.

This same experiment was used in 7 patients with hemiplegic migraine in whom paresthesiae and incoordination of the upper limb (including the hand) developed with each SP freeze and disappeared with each thaw. In 3 patients, floating scotomata (colored or otherwise) were reproduced with each freeze and cancelled with each thaw. A further 3 patients experienced a reproduction of their customary migrainic hallucinations on freezing, which again disappeared on thawing. Although I am not a neurologist, the above experiment suggests that the sympathetic plays an important role in the central phenomena which accompany attacks of classical migraine.

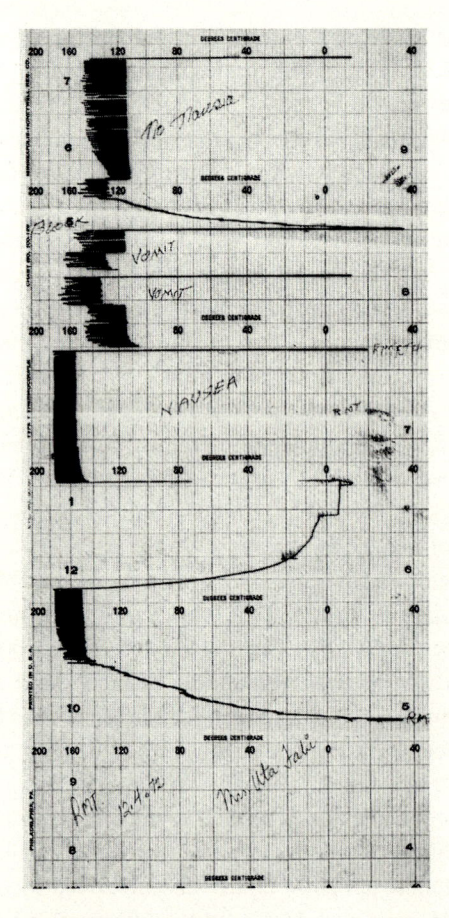

Fig. 4. The machine has drawn a chart of temperature and time. Vertical space between horizontal lines represents 20 sec. Temperature hovers at $-160\,°C$. Stellate block was done before the last (top) freeze.

Animal Experiments

Suspecting that the effect of freezing extended beyond the artery, the external carotid artery of dogs was frozen at $-140°C$ with the probe tip in contact with the artery. Following this procedure, the artery became solid and brittle, resembling a piece of macaroni, and was pulseless. When the freeze was stopped, the artery thawed out within about 2 min, assumed a

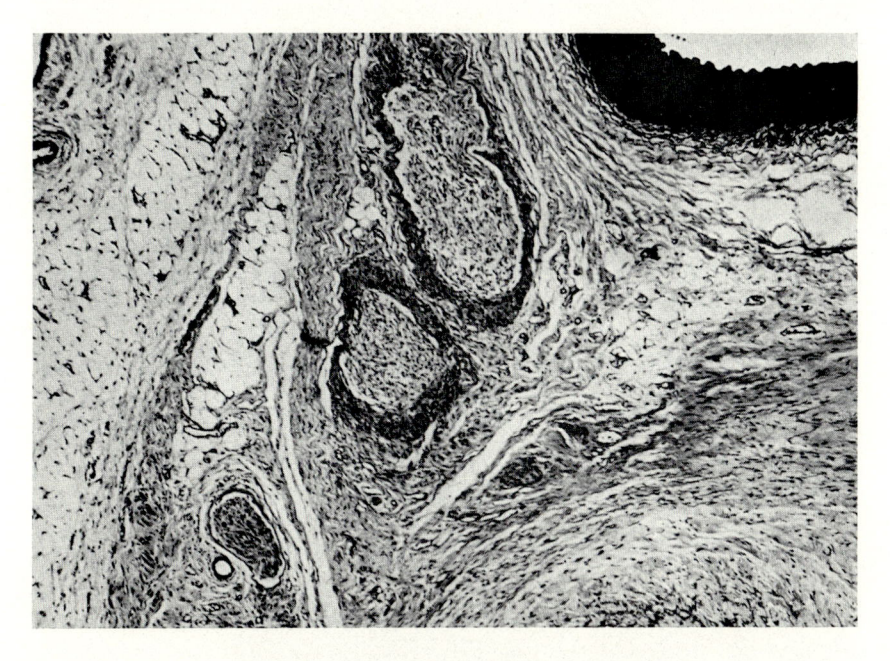

Fig. 5. 19-day dog. Florid granular inflammation outside artery, though only artery itself was frozen. Nerve bundles show inflammatory disorganization and thickened perineurium. Picture resembles periarteritis nodosum in the human. Artery upper right is intact.

blush and resumed pulsation. The animals seemed to be unaffected and were able to eat their dinner the same night.

When the dogs were sacrificed, the sections sent to Dr. K. THORNTON, our pathologist, included not only the artery but a block of surrounding tissue, because we were looking for some changes outside the artery. Figure 5 shows the 19-day dog. The artery is upper right and is intact. Paraarterial nerve bundles outside the artery, as far as 3 mm or more, show an inflammatory disorganization within the nerve bundle, a thickened perineurium and a florid granular inflammation extending some distance outside the artery. Dr. THORNTON stated that the picture is identical with that of periarteritis nodosum in the human.

The blood within the artery becomes lysed during the freeze. Most of the arteries in the body will survive freezing provided they are not frozen too long or at too low a temperature. It is therefore to be expected that arteries, because of the fast warm blood flow, will remain intact and viable despite

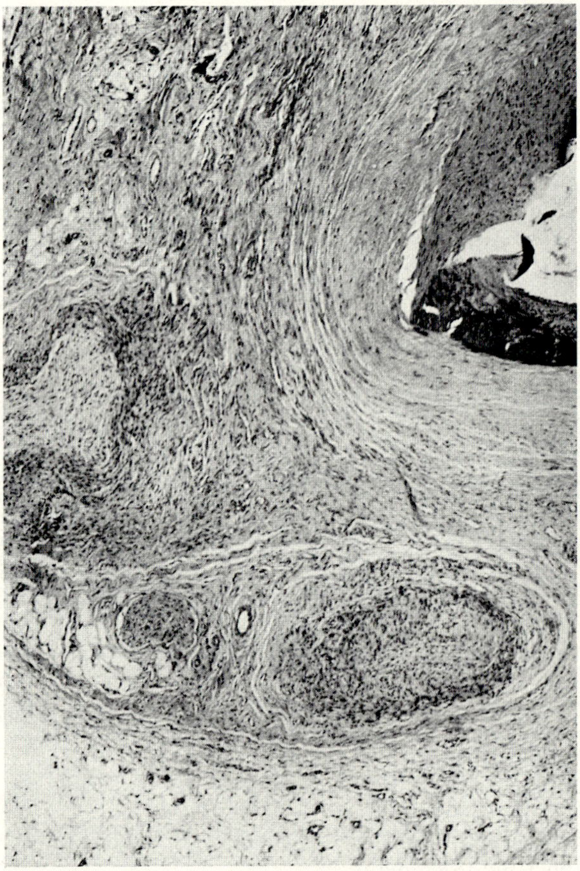

Fig. 6. 42-day dog. Artery upper right. Large nerve bundle in center of picture is degenerated. Perarterial inflammation has been replaced by fibroblasts.

the freeze but it has been shown that this is not always the case. Figure 6 shows a 42-day dog and here an inflammatory reaction has been replaced by a fibroblastic change (the artery is seen with an artefact, top left). A large nerve bundle in the center of the picture is degenerated.

It is of interest that this reaction outside the artery occurred in spite of the fact that the vessel was lifted up on a hook and the probe applied directly to the vessel. No freezing took place outside the artery. The interpretation of these pictures remains open to conjecture but there is a likelihood that cryosurgery may produce a peripheral sympathectomy.

The Transantral Approach

The transantral approach has been used in cases where cluster headache was not controlled for more than a very short time by intranasal cryosurgery. In a few cases of cluster headache, some dating back as far as 1969, this approach has produced a permanent satisfactory result. Within the last 2 years or so this technique was used almost exclusively on about 100 cases and proved to be probably less successful than the intranasal procedure. Nevertheless, it has a place. 3 recent cases of extreme cluster headache with no remissions were treated with 'both barrels of the shot gun'. This means that the intranasal procedure was used first under local anesthesia and then 2 or 3 days later, the transantral procedure was used with the patient asleep. So far these cases have done very well.

The approach is familiar to every otolaryngologist. The Caldwell-Luc approach is used, and the pterygoid space is entered through the back wall of the antrum. The maxillary artery is picked up on a blunt hook and clipped with a stainless steel clip. The artery is then followed towards the nose until the 'bag of worms' near the nose in the SP fossa is reached. Here the ganglion can often be seen by lifting the blood vessels forward. The whole complex is frozen with a 4.7-mm cryosurgical probe for 2 min at $-130°C$.

The transantral approach has not proved to be the perfect surgical answer for cryosurgery in the SP fossa. It has, however, a definite place as a reinforcing procedure where intranasal freezing has produced only a temporary result. Today, I can point to a few cases of severe cluster headache in which this approach has been successful for several years. Inevitably the transantral approach will leave a numbness in the fifth nerve distribution which may take more than a year to recover. This is an unpleasant side-effect, particularly if the patient has not achieved a good result in terms of his cluster headache.

Complications

(1) Temporary paresis of the frontalis muscle has occurred following freezing of the superficial temporal vessel. In no case has this persisted.

(2) Visual blurring has occurred many times during each freeze and has for the most part consisted of a misty spot in the peripheral field of vision, like looking through spectacles marred by a finger print.

(3) Diplopia has occurred in quite a few cases particularly in the early ones. This is usually a third nerve phenomenon and has been alarming but has, to my knowledge, always recovered and I know of no patient who retained a surgical diplopia.

(4) The sense of smell has been destroyed in several cases. The cause is mysterious because the lethal zone surrounding the small probe, well behind the olfactory area, would not be expected to injure the sense of smell, but sometimes it does. It is therefore important that the probe be buried in bone, either in the substance of the turbinate (far left, fig. 2) or in the ethmoid position (center, fig. 2) but definitely not in the position in which the probe is not insulated by bone (far right, fig. 2).

(5) A man of 69 became unconscious on the 3rd postoperative day, with his eyes deviated to the operated side. He recovered and subsequently reported a 25% improvement in his headache. A middle-aged nurse, about 4 days postoperatively, developed a paraplegia which recovered spontaneously and was never diagnosed.

(6) In a series of transantral procedures (over 100), one case developed an ischemic necrosis of the alveolar process. Presumably, the descending branch of the SP artery was obliterated.

In terms of complications, and always with legal implications in mind, in a procedure which is innovative, it is suggested that anyone wishing to use the cryosurgical procedure should use it as a treatment and not an operation. This means dropping the temperature in the desired SP location to the point where a reproduction of symptoms is obtained and being content with that. In such a case, the patient should be warned that recurrence is likely, and told that if they obtain months or a year of relief, the procedure can be repeated.

Postoperative Course

Postoperative pain is usually very severe and often accompanied by nausea and vomiting if these have been clinical features of the patient's attacks of headache. In other words, the procedure in the nose, on the SP target particularly, produces an attack of what might be compared to a severe migraine. At the end of 24 h this attack has usually subsided and the patient may then have continuing attacks of headache for a matter of weeks or months depending upon the severity of the thermal trauma and the accuracy of the probe in the SP area. These patients are told that the results of the procedure cannot be assessed for about 6 months. However, usually, whether or not a case is going to be a success or otherwise can be determined after about 3 months.

Summary

The use of cryosurgery applied to the sphenopalatine area (artery and ganglion) plus the superficial temporal and occipital branches of the external carotid artery has proven worthwhile in a majority of patients in whom this procedure has been used since 1968. Experience includes almost 700 procedures in more than 500 patients who have answered to follow-up. The procedure is not a major operation, is *repeatable* and, until the ideal drug is discovered, offers a better than average chance for definite improvement in vascular headache.

References

1 SLUDER, G.: Concerning some headaches and eye disorders of nasal origin (Mosby St. Louis 1918).
2 WOLFSON, R.J.; CUTT, R.A.; ISHIYAMA, E., and MYERS, D.: Cryosurgery for Ménière's disease. Laryngoscope *78:* 632–642 (1968).
3 LLOYD, J.W.; BARNARD, J.O.W., and GLYNN, C.J.: Cryoanalgesia – a new approach to pain relief. Lancet *ii:* 932–934 (1976).
4 OZENBERGER, J.M.: Cryosurgery in chronic rhinitis. Laryngoscope *80:* 723–734 (1970).
5 SAXENA, P.R. and VLAAM-SCHLUTER, G.M. DE: Role of some biogenic substances in migraine and relevant mechanism in antimigraine action of ergotamine. Studies in an experimental model for migraine. Headache *13:* 142–163 (1974).
6 COOK, N.: Cryosurgery of migraine. Headache *12:* 143–150 (1973).

Dr. N.C. COOK, 915 Terrace Avenue, *Victoria, V8S3V2* (Canada)

Stereotactic Treatment of Head and Neck Pain

PHILIP L. GILDENBERG

Division of Neurosurgery, The University of Texas, Texas Medical Center, Houston, Tex.

Contents

Introduction	102
Human Stereotactic Surgery	103
Stereotactic Procedures for Treatment of Pain	104
Stimulation Produced Analgesia	107
Clinical Indications	110
Cancer Pain	110
Thalamic Syndrome	112
Trigeminal Neuralgia	113
Anesthesia Dolorosa	114
Postherpetic Neuralgia	115
Atypical Facial Neuralgia	115
Headache	115
References	116

Introduction

The concept of stereotactic surgery was first introduced in animals by HORSLEY and CLARKE [36] in 1908. They devised an apparatus which could be precisely attached to the head of an experimental animal in such a way that the base of the apparatus lay in a plane parallel to the base of the animal skull. The apparatus was aligned by means of earplugs so that a second reference plane passing through the external auditory canals could be defined at right angles to the basal plane. The midsagittal plane lay in the midline at right angles to these two planes. Thus, three reference planes were defined in a precise relationship to the skull. It was possible by means of an electrode carrier to position the tip of an electrode at any desired point in space within the brain in relation to the three reference planes, for example, 3 mm anterior to the interaural plane, 2 mm to the right of the midline and 6 mm above the basal plane, so that only one point would correspond to these coordinates. An atlas was made by accurately sectioning brains of animals, usually at planes parallel to the interaural plane. The variability between a given set of coordinates and a desired structure was determined by measuring a number of sectioned brains of experimental animals so that one could anticipate with reasonable probability in which anatomical structure the tip of the electrode lay at a given set of coordinates.

Thus, if the intention was to put the tip of the electrode into a particular nucleus, by consulting the atlas, the coordinates for that structure, that is, the distance from the reference planes, could be obtained. The electrode carrier could then be positioned to bring the tip of the electrode to those coordinates and consequently to lie within the desired intracerebral structure.

However, this system did not work in the human. Because of the great difference in the shapes of human skulls and the tremendous variability between the reference planes and any given structure within the brain, it was not possible to insert the tip of the electrode with sufficient anatomical accuracy to utilize this same system in patients. Although an animal experiment could always be repeated in hopes of more accurate placements of an electrode, this luxury could not be afforded in patients where the accuracy of each electrode insertion was essential.

Human Stereotactic Surgery

It was not until 1946, when SPIEGEL et al. [87] evolved a system utilizing reference planes based on landmarks within the brain, that stereotactic surgery could be applied to the human. They performed a pneumoencephalogram to outline the third ventricle. The landmarks they originally used were the pineal body and the foramen of Monro to define the basal plane, a second plane at right angles passing through the pineal body, and the midsagittal plane. From these three reference planes measurements were made [84]. Since that time, it has become more customary to use a line between the indentations of the third ventricle representing the anterior and posterior commissures as the basal plane, a plane at right angles through the posterior commissure as the second plane, and the midsagittal plane. Also the use of Pantopaque ventriculography [85, 88] or Conray ventriculography [70, 71] makes it unnecessary to perform a pneumoencephalogram, so that patients tolerate the procedure better.

One of the first uses of stereotactic surgery when it was developed by SPIEGEL and WYCIS [83–85] 30 years ago was the treatment of pain which could not be treated by any other means. Previously cordotomy had been an accepted procedure to treat intractable pain of the body and extremities, particularly in patients with cancer, but there had been no acceptable means of interrupting fibers conducting pain sensation from the face and head. The major contribution of stereotaxis to pain surgery at that time was to introduce a treatment for head and neck pain which did not require surgical exposure in order to incise pain tracts lying very close to vital structures within the brain stem. Although those tracts had been surgically interrupted prior to that time [54, 100], the mortality and morbidity of conventional surgery usually made it impractical, particularly in patients already debilitated by poor nutrition from metastatic disease. Procedures which involved treating head and neck pain by section of the trigeminal root or Gasserian ganglion were complicated by a significant incidence of anesthesia dolorosa, which was often as severe as the original pain which had been treated.

Stereotactic Procedures for Treatment of Pain

The first SPIEGEL and WYCIS [83] paper involving treatment of pain concerns a 45-year-old man who had constant paroxysmal left face pain secondary to a thalamic syndrome. Bilateral stereotactic mesencephalotomy resulted in pain relief for 4.5 months but was complicated by persistent diplopia. With that report, the role of stereotactic surgery in the treatment of face pain was firmly demonstrated.

The recurrence of pain in that patient theoretically demonstrates that face and head pain, as well as pain elsewhere in the body, is transmitted via several different pathways, and each must be considered in a treatment program.

The classical pathway for face and head pain, the neoquintothalamic tract, which is part of the lemniscal system, involves peripheral innervation entering the brain stem via the trigeminal nerve and descending to synapse in the spinal root of the trigeminal ganglion. The second order neurons decussate and ascend in the medial lemniscus to the ventroposteromedial nucleus of the thalamus, where they again synapse with third order neurons projecting via the internal capsule to the inferior portion of the postcentral gyrus [18, 96]. It was that pathway that SPIEGEL and WYCIS interrupted at the level of the mesencephalon. However, the interruption of that pathway causes a persistent analgesia or hypesthesia of the face and may sometimes produce painful dysesthesia of the area denervated [15, 85].

The paleospinoreticulothalamic and paleoquintoreticulothalamic pathways are part of the extralemniscal system and take origin from collaterals which leave the neospinothalamic and neoquintothalamic pathways in the reticular formation and ascend via a multisynaptic system to the intralaminar and centrum medianum areas of the thalamus. The theoretical consideration is that the return of pain may be due to messages sent via this more primitive pain system, which has been implicated in poorly localized so-called visceral type of pain. This consideration led to the possibility that pain might be relieved by interruption of this more diffuse system without causing the analgesia and potential dysesthesia which may accompany neospinothalamic lesions. Stereotactic surgery made it possible to identify and safely interrupt this pathway as well.

Indeed, stereotactic lesions have been made in the area just below the thalamus to interrupt the paleoreticulothalamic pathway (basal thalamotomy), in the intralaminar area, and in the periaqueductal gray [7, 20, 21, 43–45, 52, 64, 68, 77, 85, 86, 88, 89, 93, 98]. It has also been reported [13] that pain has been successfully treated by stereotactic lesions in the pulvinar, which likewise may belong to this system.

Basal thalamotomy, however, does not appear to be merely selective interruption of the paleospinoreticulothalamic or paleoquintoreticulothalamic tract. Included in the area of the lesion may be HASSLER's Vcpc nucleus [31, 79] and the nucleus limitans [7]. Occasionally the external part of the parafascicularis nucleus and the inferior portion of the centrum medianum may be involved, although the former belongs to the same extralemniscal system as the intralaminar nuclei.

In an interesting study of cutaneous sensibility before and after basal thalamotomy for the treatment of intractable pain in 10 patients, changes in light touch were found generally confined to the area from which pain had been alleviated [7]. The authors accept this finding as evidence for a reciprocal gate control system at that level. The gate theory indicates that nonpainful stimulation may inhibit pain sensation at spinal and possibly brain stem levels (the theory upon which transcutaneous and dorsal column stimulation are based) [54]. It appears that painful sensation may reciprocally inhibit tactile sensation. These authors further theorize that the dual projection of lemniscal and extralemniscal pathways to the thalamus obscures this somatosensory inhibition, but when one of the pathways is interrupted by stereotactic surgery, this inhibition can be expressed. It is curious that such inhibition of tactile sensation can be expressed even though the pain sensation is no longer projected to conscious levels.

Head and neck pain may cause considerable emotional distress which makes the patient even less able to tolerate the pain. This is particularly true of patients with disfiguring carcinomas involving the face and head. Tumors involving the mouth or nasal cavity may likewise cause distress to the patient when he attempts to eat, and the attendant malnutrition may adversely affect the pain and the patient's condition in general.

It is possible to significantly alter these affective aspects of head and neck pain by interruption of the pathways between the dorsomedian nucleus of the thalamus and the frontal lobes [17, 65, 78]. This is the same pathway that has been attacked in classical prefrontal lobotomy [26]. It was discovered early that stereotactic lesions placed in the dorsomedian nucleus produce similar beneficial effects on pain as prefrontal lobotomy, but without the mental deterioration associated with lobotomy [33, 45, 63, 90]. However, other authors have not been as successful in obtaining permanent pain relief by this means, and prefer to combine the dorsomedian lesions with lesions in the specific or nonspecific pain projecting areas of the thalamus [97].

Lesions may also be produced to interrupt the limbic system or the connection between the thalamus and limbic system in order to treat the affective response to pain and the stressful reaction to having chronic pain. Targets for such stereotactic surgery include the anterior nucleus of the thalamus, the cingulum [10, 19, 22, 23] or the centrum medianum [24, 33, 40, 90, 98]. Patients in whom such lesions have been created respond similarly to those who have had interruptions of the prefrontal pathways for the treatment of pain.

Thus, three different opportunities are available to treat severe intractable pain of the head and neck, by interrupting different pathways alone or in combination with stereotactic surgery.

Interruption of the neoquintothalamic system results in analgesia and a loss of pain appreciation. After such lesions, patients may have relief of their intractable pain, but have also lost pain perception. This is more likely to provide immediate relief of pain and insensibility to pain, but may be attended with distressing dysesthesias. Also, when this pathway alone is interrupted, the recurrence of chronic aching pain may occur several months or years later.

Interruption of the paleoquintoreticulothalamic pathways in or just below the thalamus frequently eliminates chronic aching pain but without the production of analgesia or risk of dysesthesias. Although the possibility of immediate success with severe somatic pain such as cancer pain is not quite as good, once obtained, the chance of long-lasting pain relief is perhaps somewhat better. Patients with such lesions report alleviation of their chronic intractable pain, but do not lose the ability to perceive acute pain or a painful stimulus.

The third possibility for interruption of pain pathways by stereotactic surgery involves making a lesion in the dorsomedian nucleus or limbic system to alter the affective response to chronic pain. These patients may appear much improved, require much less medication, sleep well, and be able to participate in social activities. When asked, they may report, however, that the pain is just as severe as ever, but that 'it just doesn't bother me anymore'.

Because of the high incidence of recurrence of pain after stereotactic interruption of pathways in or about the thalamus (or any other pain-relieving procedure, for that matter), it is frequently advantageous to interrupt more than one of the pathways associated with the perception of pain. This is particularly the case in patients with cancer of the head and neck who may suffer from pain as a direct result of invasion of sensitive tissue by the tumor and who may have a great deal of anxiety and stress associated with their disfiguring and eventually terminal condition. Since the procedure is done under local anesthesia with the patient awake in order to test physiologically and clinically the location and extent of the lesion, one might first make a lesion in the extralemniscal basal or intralaminar area of the thalamus. If this does not afford sufficient pain relief, the lesion can be extended laterally to include the medial lemniscus. In those patients whose emotional status warrants, the lesion can likewise be extended medially and anteriorly to the anterior area of the dorsomedian nucleus to treat the affective aspects of the patient's symptoms as well.

Stimulation Produced Analgesia

As early as 1969, REYNOLDS [66] reported that focal brain stem stimulation in periaqueductal gray and the periventricular area of the rat could produce analgesia. This was confirmed by MAYER *et al.* [51] in 1971, who noted that stimulation-produced analgesia (SPA) can occur with no loss of acuity for other sensory modalities. At higher voltages such stimulation was sometimes associated with hyperresponsiveness to light touch. SPA appears to be a specific analgesic response and is not the same as self-stimulation reward behavior. Analgesia by stimulation of the periventricular and periaqueductal areas has since been verified in the rat [9, 41, 42, 47–49, 53, 60, 67], monkey [28, 76], cat [61] and man [2, 29, 50, 56, 69, 70, 72].

Evidence that stimulation produced analgesia is a specific antinociceptive effect and is not a generalized emotional, motivational or attentional deficit resides in the observation that it often results in a restricted peripheral field of analgesia [48, 51, 82]. Thus, noxious stimuli in some portions of the body may be ignored, whereas the same stimuli applied elsewhere elicit normal defensive responses. The animals behave normally during the application of the stimulation. In man there may be no behavioral, motivational or subjective response to stimulation at analgesic doses [2, 5, 37, 69, 72]. Other sensory modalities are intact and there is normal response to light touch and other motivational behaviors are not interrupted [51, 60, 70, 82]. The analgesia may outlast the stimulation by several hours [48, 51, 53, 70, 72].

This method has been employed clinically for treatment of intractable pain, including the head and neck, by RICHARDSON and AKIL [70, 72], MEYERSON and BOETHIUS [56] and ADAMS [2]. A four contact electrode is inserted stereotactically into an area near the third ventricle. In the first stage of the procedure, the leads are allowed to protrude through the scalp so that different combinations of the four electrode sites might be stimulated in an attempt to alleviate the patient's intractable pain. If and when it is found that satisfactory relief can be obtained in this fashion, the system is internalized. The external leads are removed and the proper pair of electrodes is connected via subcutaneous leads to a small radio receiver which lies subcutaneously at some convenient location, usually just below the clavicle. A small battery-operated radio transmitter, which the patient can hold in his hand and adjust, is connected to an antenna which is taped over the implanted radio receiver. Sufficient energy can be transmitted in this fashion so that the internalized portion requires no power supply of its own. The patient can adjust the voltage himself so that he may provide an adequate stimulus as often as needed for pain relief. Relief outlasts the stimulus by many hours, and patients need use the stimulator only intermittently. Curiously, although analgesia can be induced in experimental animals, such as the rat, cat and monkey, it cannot consistently be demonstrated in man, even when successful alleviation of chronic intractable pain occurs.

Patients who have been treated with such chronic stimulating devices include patients with pain due to cancer of the head and neck [2, 72].

Observations made on stimulation of brain stem structures in man for the relief of clinical intractable pain of all parts of the body, including the head and face, closely parallel animal observations [1, 2, 29, 56, 69, 70, 72]. Such stimulation can alleviate pain syndromes regardless of physical etiology, anatomical distribution, or the extent of the body involved. As in animal studies, analgesia in man outlasts the actual period of brain stimulation, sometimes making it necessary for the stimulator to be employed for only brief periods several times a day. Often pain relief is observed without the demonstrable analgesia on testing for pin-stick sensation. There is no particular sensation associated with stimulation-produced analgesia, but higher voltage stimulation of the same areas may produce a feeling of distress or warmth. The analgesia is particularly potent in midline structures and somewhat more on the side of the body contralateral to stimulation than ipsilateral. The pain relief occurs as readily from sites in the head and neck as from peripheral portions of the body.

Stimulation-produced analgesia bears many resemblances to morphine-produced analgesia. Both can be partially blocked by naloxone [1, 6, 46]. Tolerance develops to stimulation-produced analgesia so that patients must be instructed to employ it only intermittently [70, 72]. Animals that are made tolerant to morphine simultaneously develop tolerance to stimulation-produced analgesia, although the reverse is not true [47]. It has been hypothesized that stimulation-produced analgesia may result from the release of an endogenous morphine-like substance, possibly endorphine, which then acts at opiate receptor sites in the brain stem [4, 46, 48, 70, 71].

Although the periventricular and periaqueductal areas are the only regions the stimulation of which results in analgesia in experimental animals, there had been even earlier reports of pain relief in man by stimulation of other areas. The first such report actually antedates stimulation-produced analgesia by 20 years. HEATH and MICKLE [32] stimulated the septal area in humans with intractable pain. This site corresponds to a reward area in the rat, and the intention was to see if any such reward sensation existed in the human and, if so, whether it might alleviate some of the emotional distress associated with terminal cancer. It was found, however, that such stimulation alleviated the pain but did not provide any apparent sensation of reward, as later confirmed by others [27].

ADAMS and HOSOBUCHI [2, 3, 38] stimulated the internal capsule or the primary thalamic relay nuclei of the thalamus to treat successfully pain secondary to lesions which might deprive the individual of some sensory input, such as thalamic syndrome, traumatic painful paraplegia or phantom limb pain.

Clinical Indications

Unfortunately, much of the literature concerning the stereotactic treatment of pain does not specify whether patients in the various series had head and neck pain. Other authors may separate pain by areas of the body, but then group all patients together when considering their results.

Cancer Pain

There are several conditions causing pain of the head and face which lend themselves particularly well to treatment by stereotactic surgery. Pertinent among these is cancer pain. Not only are tumors of the head and face frequently not completely resectable because of the complex anatomy of the region, but the tissues involved are quite sensitive to pain. This is coupled with the extreme discomfort and distress caused by interference with eating, speaking and breathing. In addition, the attendant psychological distress in patients with disfiguring tumors of the face frequently causes such patients to tolerate their pain very poorly, and makes pain relief critical. Indeed, patients whose pain is successfully relieved may benefit by the associated improvement in eating and nutrition, which may add significantly to the duration and quality of survival.

When patients with pain of any etiology are taken as a group, regardless of the location of the stereotactic lesion in the brain, if the patient lives long enough, there is a better than 50% chance that the pain will recur. Consequently, patients with pain secondary to malignancy have a greater possibility of permanent pain relief than other patients with chronic pain.

There are several valid targets for making stereotactic lesions for the treatment of head and neck pain secondary to tumor. Various authors have reported on different targets with similar chances for success or complication.

The target first employed in the stereotactic treatment of head and face pain secondary to malignancy is in the intralaminar nuclei just where the extralemniscal fibres enter the base of the thalamus, so-called basal thalamotomy [20, 21, 64, 85, 86, 88, 89]. Reports have been of 70% or more of cancer patients obtaining satisfactory pain relief from a lesion in this area. This target site has the advantage that patients do not demonstrate complete insensitivity. It is in an area where the lesion might easily be extended to the lemniscal tracts or medial thalamus, and the lesion is above those brain stem cranial nuclei which might produce complications, particularly involving extraocular movements. Some authors [7, 64] routinely make somewhat larger lesions to include the lemniscal fibers as they enter the ventroposteromedial nucleus, or possibly the centrum medianum nucleus as well.

Other neurosurgeons prefer to make the lesions slightly lower in the mesencephalon, where the various pain tracts run more compactly and both lemniscal and extralemniscal tracts can be interrupted with a small lesion [57, 75, 83, 97]. The occurrence of analgesia or even anesthesia dolorosa with lesions in this area appears to be somewhat higher than lesions in the thalamus, and there is a risk of the lesion involving the uppermost oculomotor fibers to cause an extraocular palsy, usually of little clinical significance. The authors who advocate mesencephalotomy, however, feel that the chance of pain relief is greater and worth the slight additional risk.

The first report of pain relief from a centrum medianum lesion occurred in 1949 (prior to the first report of similar lesions by stereotactic surgery) after a thromboembolic extension of a thalamic syndrome [33]. Some authors prefer the centrum medianum as their target to treat pain of malignancy [24, 40]. SUGITA [90], who prefers to make lesions in the centrum medianum and part of the dorsomedian nucleus, reports that almost all of his patients with head and neck pain secondary to malignancy obtain a significant amount of pain relief. LEKSELL [24, 40] performs his stereotactic surgery with an apparatus that focuses gamma radiation on a point which can be aligned with stereotactic coordinates to involve the centrum medianum. Although most of his patients have pain in the body rather than the head, and although he reports only a 40% incidence of pain relief, the technique is of some interest because it is completely noninvasive.

Stereotactic trigeminal tractotomy involves a suboccipital approach to introduce an electrode into the descending tract of the trigeminal nerve [14, 25, 34, 35, 80, 81, 95]. Stimulation during surgery has verified the onion skin distribution of fibers in this tract [80, 81] and assists in making a discrete lesion involving only those areas involved with pain. Consequently, this procedure may be somewhat better for patients with more localized head or face pain. Analgesia is obtained as after a cordotomy, and almost universally good pain relief in cancer patients is reported.

Stereotactic insertion of chronic stimulating electrodes into the periventricular gray likewise is advocated in selected patients with widespread pain of malignancy [72]. Although results have been satisfactory in most patients, the pain relief may be only partial and tolerance to constant stimulation or narcotics used in conjunction with stimulation may be a problem. Consequently, these patients must be quite critically selected.

Thalamic Syndrome

Patients with pain secondary to the thalamic syndrome of Dejerine-Roussy frequently have severe constant pain and hyperpathia involving the face as well as other parts of the body or extremities on one side [15].

The thalamic syndrome as originally described involves a hemiplegia or hemiparesis, sensory disturbance over all or a large part of the body contralateral to the lesion, including astereognosis and sometimes choreoathetoid movements of the extremities. There is often a superficial hemianesthesia which may be replaced by a cutaneous hyperesthesia or profound dysesthesia [16]. Although the incidence of such a syndrome after stroke is fairly uncommon, probably not exceeding 1 in 1,500, it can be extremely persistent and disabling, and defies usual methods of pain control. The infarction which most frequently results in the thalamic syndrome affects primarily the ventral and lateral portions of the thalamus, most often implicating the thalamogeniculate artery to the lateral thalamic nuclei, involving the ventral posterolateral and ventral posteromedial nuclei of the thalamus [15].

No procedure has been found to be consistently helpful in treating the thalamic syndrome, undoubtedly because of the variability of the lesions causing this condition [15]. Such pain defies treatment by analgesics or any other conventional pain therapy. It is only with stereotactic surgery that it has been possible to alleviate pain for many of these patients, and, even at best, success has been reported inconsistently.

Stereotactic operations for thalamic pain overall provide early relief in 75% of patients. However, 60% of patients have a return of pain between 6 months and 1 year later [15]. Spiegel *et al.* [85, 88] reported some success after making a basal thalamic lesion, presumably enlarging the stroke-induced lesion which had caused the original pain, but fewer than half of the patients thus treated had significant relief. Other neurosurgeons produced stereotactic lesions in the posteroventrolateral, or posteroventromedial nuclei to treat the pain of the thalamic syndrome [30]. Theoretically, it is the damaged remaining portion of these nuclei which produces the aberrant firing which is perceived as pain, so that destruction of the remainder of the nuclei might alleviate that pain. A review of several series reveals significant lasting relief in 11 of 17 patients treated with lesions in this nuclear group, most of whom had some component of pain in the face [11, 30, 59, 92].

Some neurosurgeons [57, 74, 75, 83] treat thalamic syndrome pain by making a lesion at midbrain levels in order to 'deafferent' the involved area of the thalamus, theorizing that the incoming information is distorted so that the patient interprets it as pain at the conscious level. SPIEGEL and WYCIS [85, 102) reported a total of 16 patients with pain of thalamic syndrome origin (the largest series in the literature), many of whom had involvement of the face and head. 3 patients were completely unrelieved of their pain by mesencephalotomy and 4 others had a complete return of pain. 2 had partial return of pain in 1–5 months, and 2 patients died too soon after surgery for long-term follow-up, leaving only 5 patients with prolonged significant relief of pain.

Trigeminal Neuralgia

Although percutaneous electrode coagulation of the trigeminal ganglia and rootlets for the treatment of trigeminal neuralgia or other face pain is not truly a stereotactic procedure employing a three-dimensional coordinate system or guiding apparatus, it has so much in common that a brief note should be included here. It employs the same temperature-controlled type of needle electrode, stimulation and recording techniques for verifying the position of the electrode, and the production of a heating lesion by radio frequency current as in stereotactic procedures.

This procedure took origin in 1931 when KIRSCHNER [39] coagulated the trigeminal ganglion with an electrosurgical unit, but abandoned the procedure after several hundred cases because of complications resulting from the uncontrolled spread of heat to adjacent cranial nerves and brain stem structures. When the development of stereotactic surgery gave impetus to the design of radio frequency generators with precise temperature control, the technique was reintroduced in 1965 by SWEET and WEPSIC [91, 101].

Reports of over 2,000 such procedures indicate that this technique has an extremely low rate of major and minor complications, certainly significantly less than surgical techniques, with results which are almost comparable [55, 58, 62, 73, 91, 94, 99].

Most authors use the technique whereby a needle is inserted 2–3 cm lateral to the canthus of the lip on the involved side. A finger within the cheek assures that the oral cavity is not penetrated as the needle is advanced through the foramen ovale under X-ray guidance. Control can be obtained either through submental vertex X-ray views or by using landmarks on lateral X-rays. When the tip of the electrode enters the trigeminal cistern, a flow of cerebrospinal fluid is seen. Either a temperature-monitoring electrode or steel wire electrode is then introduced through the needle to lie within the fibers of the trigeminal nerve. Rootlets from each division lie at successively deeper penetration with mandibular division fibers just within the foramen ovale and the ophthalmic division lying 12–14 mm deep. Placement of the electrode can be verified by stimulating at very low voltages prior to the production of a graded radio frequency lesion.

The mortality rate is extremely low, one death having been reported in the literature. Unwanted corneal anesthesia occurred in an average of 4.9% in eight published series [99], as compared to 6–10% in open surgical techniques. Painful dysesthesias occurred in an average of 2.4% with radio frequency lesions, as compared to an average of 26.4% in two large surgical series. Consequently, one must consider this semistereotactic procedure to be the ganglionectomy of choice in trigeminal neuralgia refractory to other forms of treatment.

SCHVARCZ [80] reported using stereotactic trigeminal tractotomy with good results for the treatment of trigeminal neuralgia in 11 patients who were refractory to medical treatment, and TODD et al. [95] also reported one patient with tic successfully treated with tractotomy. Although it seems difficult to justify making a lesion centrally when one might control this condition with a peripheral lesion, these results are quite encouraging in the absence of any significant complications.

Anesthesia Dolorosa

One of the dreaded complications following surgical section of the trigeminal nerve or its roots is that of anesthesia dolorosa. Previously, this frustrating condition had defied almost all attempts at treatment. However, several stereotactic procedures have offered new opportunities. Mesencephalotomy has been reported to be of some help if there is a residual dysesthesia component following an incomplete section of the trigeminal nerve [83]. SCHVARCZ [80] reported successful treatment of 3 patients with anesthesia dolorosa by stereotactic trigeminal tractotomy of the descending trigeminal tract or nucleus caudalis.

However, patients with pain of anesthesia dolorosa perhaps appear to do better with chronic stimulation than with destructive techniques. In an attempt to provide the sensation which had been interrupted, HOSOBUCHI et al. [38] implanted chronic stimulation electrodes in the posteroventral medial nucleus of the thalamus with good results in 4 patients. Although follow-up is short and experience limited, this procedure appears to be more successful than previous stereotactic methods of treating these patients with lesions in the thalamus [85].

Postherpetic Neuralgia

An additional painful disabling condition which has heretofore defied most attempts at treatment is postherpetic neuralgia in the trigeminal nerve distribution. A number of reports have appeared demonstrating consistently good results in selected patients by stereotactic trigeminal tractotomy at the cervicomedullary junction [25, 34, 80, 81]. Theoretically the virus attacks the trigeminal nerve peripherally at its ganglion or perhaps at the synapse between the first and second order neuron. The tractotomy can be made high enough to interrupt the second order neuron as it ascends toward the thalamus, thereby disassociating the involved portion of the sensory system with its central connections.

Atypical Facial Neuralgia

The final condition mentioned in the stereotactic literature concerning treatment of head and face pain is 'atypical facial neuralgia'. However, there does not appear to be uniform definition of this condition, and the results are universally unsatisfactory, provoking the conclusion that one must select these patients with great care and consideration of psychiatric factors.

Headache

It has been reported that patients with suboccipital tension type headache who are not responsive to any other means of treatment may benefit from radio frequency coagulation of the insertion of the suboccipital muscles just medial to the mastoid area. This is the same group of patients whose headaches respond dramatically to local anesthetic blocks of the same areas and who might be treated by other means such as repeated blocks of local anesthetic or phenol blocks in these areas. BLUME [12] reports a 78% significant relief of occipital headache in 114 cases in whom the radio frequency coagulation procedure was used. From his description, one might assume that these were primarily cases of muscle tension headache. Again, although this is not a stereotactic procedure, the temperature-monitored radio frequency electrode employed is directly derived from that used in stereotactic surgery.

A modality closely related to stereotactic surgery is transcutaneous stimulation. This method is based on the MELZACK and WALL pain theory [54], which suggests that a nonpainful stimulus applied peripherally tends to inhibit pain, such as may happen when one rubs an injured area. APPENZELLER [8] recently reported on the use of this device for the treatment of migraine and other headaches, claiming successful treatment in 10 of 12 migraine patients. He also reported success in 2 patients with trigeminal neuralgia, which is contrary to the experiences of most others, and 4 cases of other unspecified neuralgia. His report of success in 12 of 15 patients with tension headaches parallels my own experience, and this is an area which might be suggested for future investigation.

References

1 ADAMS, J.E.: Naloxone reversal of analgesia produced by brain stimulation in the human. Pain 2: 161–166 (1976).
2 ADAMS, J.E.: Technique and technical problems associated with implantation of neuroaugmentative devices. Appl. Neurophysiol. (in publication).
3 ADAMS, J.E.; HOSOBUCHI, Y., and FIELDS, H.L.: Stimulation of internal capsule for relief of chronic pain. J. Neurosurg. 41: 740–744 (1974).
4 AKIL, H. and LIEBESKIND, J.C.: Monoaminergic mechanisms of stimulation-produced analgesia. Brain Res. 94: 279–296 (1975).
5 AKIL, H.; MAYER, D.J. et LIEBESKIND, J.C.: Psychophysiologie – comparaison chez le rat entre l'analgésie induite par stimulation de la substance grise péri-aqueducale et l'analgésie morphinique. C. r. hebd. Séanc. Acad. Sci., Paris 274: 3603–3605 (1972).
6 AKIL, H. and RICHARDSON, D.E.: Electrophysiological correlates of stimulation produced analgesia, morphine analgesia, and their blockade by naloxone. Proc. Soc. Neurosci. Annual Meeting, St. Louis 1974, p. 114.
7 ALBE-FESSARD, D.; DONDEY, M.; NICOLAIDIS, S., and LEBEAU, J.: Remarks concerning the effect of diencephalic lesions on pain and sensitivity with special reference to lemniscally mediated control of noxious afferences. Confinia neurol. 32: 174–184 (1970).
8 APPENZELLER, O. und ATKINSON, R.: Transkutane Nervenreizung zur Behandlung der Migraine und anderer Kopfschmerzen. Münch. med. Wschr. 117: 1953–1954 (1975).
9 BALGURA, S. and RALPH, T.: The analgesic effect of electrical stimulation of the diencephalon and mesencephalon. Brain Res. 60: 369–379 (1973).
10 BALLANTINE, H.T., jr.; CASSIDY, W.L.; FLANAGAN, N.D., and MARINO, R., Jr.: Stereotaxic anterior cingulotomy for neuropsychiatric illness and intractable pain. J. Neurosurg. 26: 488–495 (1967).
11 BETTAG, W. und YOSHIDA, T.: Stereotaktische Schmerzoperationen. Acta neurochir. 8: 299–317 (1960).
12 BLUME, H.G.: Radio frequency denaturation in occipital pain. A new approach in 114 cases. Adv. Pain Res. Ther. 1: 691–698 (1976).
13 COOPER, I.S.: A surgical investigation of the clinical physiology of the LP-pulvinar complex in man. J. neurol. Sci. 18: 89–110 (1973).
14 CRUE, B.L.; TODD, E.M., and CARREGAL, E.J.: Percutaneous radio frequency stereotactic tractotomy; in CRUE Pain and suffering, pp. 69–79 (Thomas, Springfield 1970).

15 DAVIS, R.A. and STOKES, J.W.: Neurosurgical attempts to relieve thalamic pain. Surgery Gynec. Obstet. *123:* 371–384 (1966).
16 DEJERINE, J. et ROUSSY, G.: Le syndrome thalamique. Revue neurol. *14:* 521–532 (1906).
17 DYNES, J.B. and POPPEN, J.L.: Lobotomy for intractable pain. J. Am. med. Ass. *140:* 15–19 (1949).
18 EYZAGUIRRE, C. and FIDONE, S.J.: Physiology of the nervous system; 2nd ed. (Year Book, Chicago 1975).
19 FAILLACE, L.A.; ALLEN, R.P.; MCQUEEN, J.D., and NORTHRUP, B.: Cognitive deficits from bilateral cingulotomy for intractable pain in man. Dis. nerv. Syst. *32:* 171–175 (1971).
20 FAIRMAN, D.: Evaluation of results in stereotactic thalamotomy for the treatment of intractable pain. Confinia neurol. *27:* 67–70 (1966).
21 FAIRMAN, D.: Stereotactic treatment for the alleviation of intractable pain. Reassessments and limitations. Confinia neurol. *32:* 341–344 (1970).
22 FOLTZ, E.L. and WHITE, L.E., jr.: Pain 'relief' by frontal cingulotomy. J. Neurosurg. *19:* 89–100 (1962).
23 FOLTZ, E.L. and WHITE, L.E., jr.: The role of rostral cingulotomy in 'pain' relief. Int. J. Neurol. *6:* 353–373 (1968).
24 FORSTER, D.M.C.; LEKSELL, L., and MEYERSON, B.A.: Gamma-thalamotomy in intractable pain. Presented at the 5th Int. Symp. on Stereoencephalotomy, Freiburg 1970.
25 FOX, J.L.: Percutaneous trigeminal tractotomy for facial pain. Acta neurochir. *29:* 83–88 (1973).
26 FREEMAN, W. and WATTS, J.N.: Psychosurgery in the treatment of mental disorders and intractable pain (Thomas, Springfield 1950).
27 GOL, A.: Relief of pain by electrical stimulation of the septal area. J. neurol. Sci. *5:* 115–120 (1967).
28 GOODMAN, S.J. and HOLCOMBE, V.: Selective and prolonged analgesia in monkey resulting from brain stimulation; in First World Congress on Pain, p. 264 (1975).
29 GYBELS, J.; HESS, J. VAN, and PELUSO, F.: Modulation of experimentally produced pain in man by electrical stimulation of some cortical, thalamic and basal ganglia structures; in ZOTTERMAN Sensory functions of the skin in primates, with special reference to man. Wenner-Gren Center International Symposium Series (Pergamon, Oxford 1976).
30 HANKINSON, J.; PEARCE, G.W., and ROWBOTHAM, G.F.: Stereotaxic operations for the relief of pain. J. Neurol. Neurosurg. Psychiat. *23:* 352 (1960).
31 HASSLER, R. und REICHERT, T.: Klinische und anatomische Befunde bei stereotaktischen Schmerzoperationen im Thalamus. Arch. Psychiat. *200:* 92–122 (1959).
32 HEATH, R.G. and MICKLE, W.A.: Evaluation of seven years' experience with depth electrode studies in human patients; in RAMEY and O'DOHERTY Electrical studies on the unanesthetized brain, pp. 214–217 (Hoeber, New York 1960).
33 HECAEN, H.; TALAIRACH, J.; DAVID, M. et DELL, M.B.: Coagulations limitées du thalamus dans les algies du syndrome thalamique. Résultats thérapeutiques et physiologiques. Revue neurol. *81:* 917–931 (1949).
34 HITCHCOCK, E.R.: Stereotactic trigeminal tractotomy. Ann. clin. Res. *2:* 131–135 (1970).

35 HITCHCOCK, E.R. and SCHVARCZ, J.R.: Stereotactic trigeminal tractotomy for postherpetic facial pain. J. Neurosurg. *37:* 412–417 (1972).
36 HORSLEY, V. and CLARKE, R.H.: The structure and functions of the cerebellum examined by a new method. Brain *31:* 45–124 (1908).
37 HOSOBUCHI, Y.; ADAMS, J.E., and LYNCHITZ, R.: Pain relief by electrical stimulation of the central gray matter in humans. Proc. 6th Annu. Meet., Society for Neuroscience, Toronto 1976.
38 HOSOBUCHI, Y.; ADAMS, J.E., and RUTKIN, B.: Chronic thalamic stimulation for the control of facial anesthesia dolorosa. Archs Neurol. *29:* 158–161 (1973).
39 KIRSCHNER, M.: Zur Elektrochirurgie. Arch. klin. Chir. *167:* 761–768 (1931).
40 LEKSELL, L.; MEYERSON, B.A., and FORSTER, D.M.C.: Radiosurgical thalamotomy for intractable pain. Confinia neurol. *34:* 264 (1972).
41 LIEBESKIND, J.C.: Pain modulation by central nervous system stimulation; in BONICA and ALBE-FESSARD Advances in pain research and therapy, vol. 1, pp. 445–453 (Raven Press, New York 1976).
42 LIEBESKIND, J.C. and MAYER, D.J.: Somatosensory evoked responses in the mesencephalic central gray matter of the rat. Brain Res. *27:* 133–151 (1971).
43 LOGUE, V. and WATKINS, E.S.: The treatment of intractable pain by stereotaxic thalamotomy. Report to Medical Research Council, Great Britain (1962).
44 MARK, V.H. and ERVIN, F.R.: Stereotactic surgery for relief of pain; in WHITE and SWEET Pain and the neurosurgeon, pp. 843–887 (Thomas, Springfield 1969).
45 MARK, V.H.; ERWIN, F.R., and YAKOVLEV, P.I.: Stereotactic thalamotomy. Archs Neurol. *8:* 528–538 (1963).
46 MAYER, D.J.: Pain inhibition by electrical brain stimulation. Comparison to morphine. Neurosci. Res. Prog. Bull. *13:* 94–99 (1975).
47 MAYER, D.J. and HAYES, R.L.: Stimulation produced analgesia. Development of tolerance and cross-tolerance to morphine. Science *188:* 941–943 (1975).
48 MAYER, D.J. and LIEBESKIND, J.C.: Pain reduction by focal electrical stimulation of the brain. An anatomical and behavioral analysis. Brain Res. *68:* 73–93 (1974).
49 MAYER, D.J. and MURFIN, R.: Stimulation produced analgesia (SPA) and morphine analgesia (MA). Cross-tolerance from application at the same brain site. Fed. Proc. *35:* 385 (1976).
50 MAYER, D.J.; PRICE, D.D., and BECKER, D.P.: Neurophysiological characterization of the anterolateral spinal cord neurons contributing to pain perception in man. Pain *1:* 51–58 (1975).
51 MAYER, D.J.; WOLFLE, T.L.; AKIL, H.; CARDER, B., and LIEBESKIND, J.C.: Analgesia from electrical stimulation in the brain stem of the rat. Science *174:* 1351–1354 (1971).
52 MEHLER, W.R.: The posterior thalamic region in man. Confinia neurol. *27:* 18–29 (1966).
53 MELZACK, R. and MELINKOFF, D.F.: Analgesia produced by brain stimulation. Evidence of a prolonged onset period. Expl. Neurol. *43:* 369–374 (1974).
54 MELZACK, R. and WALL, P.D.: Pain mechanisms: a new theory. Science *150:* 971–979 (1965).
55 MENZEL, J.; PIOTROWSKI, W., and PENZHOLZ, H.: Long-term results of Gasserian ganglion electrocoagulation. J. Neurosurg. *42:* 140–143 (1975).
56 MEYERSON, B. and BOETHIUS, J.: Chronic percutaneous deep brain stimulation in cancer pain. Appl. Neurophysiol. (in press).

57 NASHOLD, B.S., jr.; WILSON, W.P., and SLAUGHTER, D.G.: Sterotactic midbrain lesions for central dysesthesia and phantom pain. J. Neurosurg. 30: 116–126 (1969).
58 NUGENT, G.R. and BERRY, B.: Trigeminal neuralgia treated by differential percutaneous radio frequency coagulation of the Gasserian ganglion. J. Neurosurg. 40: 517–523 (1974).
59 OBRADOR, S.; DIERSSEN, G., and CEBALLOS, R.: Consideraciones clinicas, neurologicas y anatomicas sobre el llamado dolor talamico. Acta neurol. latinoam. 3: 58–77 (1957).
60 OLIVERAS, J.-L.; BESSON, J.-M.; GUILBAUD, G., and LIEBESKIND, J.C.: Behavioral and electrophysiological evidence of pain inhibition from midbrain stimulation in the cat. Expl. Brain Res. 20: 32–44 (1974).
61 OLIVERAS, J.-L.; REDJEMI, F.; GUILBAUD, G., and BESSON, J.M.: Analgesia induced by electrical stimulation of the inferior centralis nucleus of the raphe in the cat. Pain 1: 139–145 (1975).
62 ONOFRIO, B.M.: Radio frequency percutaneous Gasserian ganglion lesions; results in 140 patients with trigeminal pain. J. Neurosurg. 42: 132–139 (1975).
63 ORTHNER, H.: Weitere klinische und anatomische Erfahrungen mit zerebralen Schmerzoperationen. Confinia neurol. 27: 71–74 (1966).
64 PAGNI, C.A. and MASPES, P.E.: The relief of intractable pain in malignant disease of the head and neck by stereotactic thalamotomy or sensory root section; in JANZEN, KEIDEL, HERZ and STEICHELE Pain, pp. 204–207 (Williams & Wilkins, Baltimore 1972).
65 POPPEN, J.L.: Prefrontal lobotomy for intractable pain. Case report. Lahey clin. Bull. 4: 205–207 (1946).
66 REYNOLDS, D.V.: Surgery in the rat during electrical analgesia induced by focal brain stimulation. Science 164: 445 (1969).
67 RHODES, D.L.: Ph.D. diss. UCLA (1975); cit. LIEBESKIND [41].
68 RICHARDSON, D.E.: Thalamotomy for intractable pain. Confinia neurol. 29: 139–145 (1967).
69 RICHARDSON, D.E. and AKIL, H.: Acute relief of intractable pain by brain stimulation in human patients. Ann. Meet. Am. Ass. Neurol. Surg. (1973).
70 RICHARDSON, D.E. and AKIL, H.: Pain reduction by electrical brain stimulation in man. 1. Acute administration in periaqueductal and periventricular sites. J. Neurosurg. 47: 178–183 (1977).
71 RICHARDSON, D.E. and AKIL, H.: Pain reduction by electrical brain stimulation in man. 2. Chronic self-administration in the periventricular gray matter. J. Neurosurg. 47: 184–194 (1977).
72 RICHARDSON, D.E. and AKIL, H.: Pain reduction by electrical stimulation in man. Long-term results of periventricular gray self-stimulation. Pain (in press).
73 RIECHERT, T.: Interim report on induction coagulation in neurosurgical treatment of chronic pain; in JANZEN, KEIDEL, HERZ and STEICHELE Pain, pp. 198–200 (Williams & Wilkins, Baltimore 1972).
74 ROEDER, F. und ORTHNER, H.: Erfahrungen mit stereotaktischen Eingriffen. III. Mitteilung. Über zerebrale Schmerzoperationen, insbesondere mediale Mesencephalotomie bei thalamischer Hyperpathie und bei Anesthesia dolorosa. Confinia neurol. 21: 51–97 (1961).

75 ROEDER, F.; ORTHNER, H., and MULLER, D.: Studies with stereotactic surgery in the Gasserian ganglion and mesencephalon in combination with other methods (additional thalamotomy); in JANZEN, KEIDEL, HERZ and STEICHELE Pain, pp. 200–202 (Williams & Wilkins, Baltimore 1972).

76 RUDA, M.; HAYES, R.L.; DUBNER, R., and PRICE, D.D.: Analgesic and electrophysiological effects of stimulation of medial mesencephalic and diencephalic structures in the primate by electrical current or narcotic microinjection. Proc. Soc. Neurosci. 2 (1976).

77 SANO, K.; YOSHIOKA, M.; OGASHIWA, M.; ISHIJIMA, B., and OHYE, C.: Thalamolaminotomy. A new operation for the relief of intractable pain. Confinia neurol. 27: 63–66 (1966).

78 SCARFF, J.E.: Unilateral prefrontal lobotomy for the relief of intractable pain and termination of narcotic addiction. Surgery Gynec. Obstet. 89: 385–392 (1949).

79 SCHALTENBRAND, G. and BAILEY, P.: Introduction to stereotaxis with an atlas of the human brain (Grune & Stratton, Thieme, New York/Stuttgart 1959).

80 SCHVARCZ, J.R.: Stereotactic trigeminal tractotomy. Confinia neurol. 37: 73–77 (1975).

81 SCHVARCZ, J.R.: Stereotactic trigeminal nucleotomy. Evaluation of 100 cases. Appl. Neurophysiol. (in press).

82 SOPER, W.Y.: Effects of analgesic midbrain stimulation on reflex withdrawal and thermal escape in the rat. J. comp. physiol. Psychol. 90: 91–101 (1976).

83 SPIEGEL, E.A. and WYCIS, H.T.: Mesencephalotomy in treatment of 'intractable' facial pain. Archs Neurol. Psychiat., Chicago 69: 1–13 (1953).

84 SPIEGEL, E.A. and WYCIS, H.T.: Stereoencephalotomy. I. Methods and stereotaxic atlas of the human brain (Grune & Stratton, New York 1952).

85 SPIEGEL, E.A. and WYCIS, H.T.: Stereoencephalotomy. II. Clinical and physiological applications (Grune & Stratton, New York 1962).

86 SPIEGEL, E.A. and WYCIS, H.T.: Present status of stereoencephalotomies for pain relief. Confinia neurol. 27: 7–17 (1966).

87 SPIEGEL, E.A.; WYCIS, H.T.; MARKS, M., and LEE, A.J.: Stereotaxic apparatus for operations on the human brain. Science 106: 349–350 (1947).

88 SPIEGEL, E.A.; WYCIS, H.T.; SZEKELY, E.G., and GILDENBERG, P.L.: Medial and basal thalamotomy in so-called intractable pain; in KNIGHTON and DUMKE Pain, pp. 503–517 (Little Brown, Boston 1966).

89 SPIEGEL, E.A.; WYCIS, H.T.; SZEKELY, E.G.; GILDENBERG, P.L., and ZANES, C.: Combined dorsomedial, intralaminar and basal thalamotomy for the relief of so-called intractable pain. J. int. Coll. Surg. 42: 160–168 (1964).

90 SUGITA, K.; MUTSUGA, N.; TAKAOKA, Y., and DOI, T.: Results of stereotaxic thalamotomy for pain. Confinia neurol. 34: 265–274 (1972).

91 SWEET, W.H. and WEPSIC, J.G.: Controlled thermocoagulation of trigeminal ganglion and rootlets for differential destruction of pain fibers. I. Trigeminal neuralgia. J. Neursurg. 40: 143–156 (1974).

92 TALAIRACH, J.; HECAEN, H.; DAVID, M.; MONNIER, M. et AJURIAGUERRA, J. DE: Recherches sur la coagulation thérapeutique des structures souscorticales chez l'homme. Revue neurol. 81: 4–24 (1949).

93 TASKER, R.R.; ROWE, I.H.; HAWRYLYSHYN, P., and ORGAN, L.W.: Computer mapping of brain stem sensory centers in man. J. Neurosurg. 44: 458–464 (1976).

94 TEW, J.M., jr. and MAYFIELD, F.H.: Trigeminal neuralgia. A new surgical approach (percutaneous electrocoagulation of the trigeminal nerve). Laryngoscope 83: 1096–1101 (1973).
95 TODD, E.M.; CRUE, B.L., and CARREGAL, E.J.A.: Posterior percutaneous tractotomy and cordotomy. Confinia neurol. 31: 106–115 (1969).
96 TRUEX, R.C. and CARPENTER, M.: Strong and Elwyn's human neuroanatomy; 5th ed. (Williams & Wilkins, Baltimore 1964).
97 VORIS, H.C. and WHISLER, W.W.: Results of stereotaxic surgery for intractable pain. Confinia neurol. 37: 86–96 (1975).
98 WATKINS, E.S.: Stereotactic thalamotomy for intractable pain. Presented at the Meeting of the Harvey Cushing Society, St. Louis 1966.
99 WEPSIC, J.G.: Complications of percutaneous surgery for pain. Clin. Neurosurg. 23: 454–464 (1976).
100 WHITE, J.C. and SWEET, W.H.: Pain. Its mechanisms and neurosurgical control (Thomas, Springfield 1955).
101 WHITE, J.C. and SWEET, W.H.: Pain and the neurosurgeon. A 40 year experience (Thomas, Springfield 1969).
102 WYCIS, H.T. and SPIEGEL, E.A.: Long-range results in the treatment of intractable pain by stereotaxic midbrain surgery. J. Neurosurg. 19: 101–107 (1962).

PHILIP L. GILDENBERG, MD, Ph.D., Professor and Chief, Division of Neurosurgery, University of Texas Medical School at Houston, 6400 West Cullen Street, *Houston, 77030* (USA)

Chronic Brain Stimulation for the Treatment of Intractable Pain

Yoshio Hosobuchi[1]

Department of Neurosurgery, University of California School of Medicine, San Francisco, Calif.

Choosing the optimal treatment for the disabling pain that may arise from lesions in the nervous system presents perplexing problems for both neurologists and neurosurgeons. Although many neurosurgeons manage this pain by the selective destruction of certain foci in the brain, these procedures are variably efficient in relieving pain and, in general, any relief that they effect is short-lived [13].

During the course of performing one such surgical procedure – a medial thalamotomy for the treatment of facial anesthesia dolorosa – we noticed that immediate relief of facial dysesthesia occurred during the electrical stimulation of the contralateral posterior ventral medialis (PVM) nucleus of the thalamus [7]. This relief remained constant while the current was on, and persisted for 2–3 min after the current was turned off. The patients experienced paresthesia that customarily occurs with stimulation of the sensory nucleus. This stimulation-induced pain relief resembled that obtained with the use of chronically implanted peripheral nerve and dorsal column stimulators, which in clinical application have succeeded in alleviating many previously tenacious pain syndromes [12].

Drawing on our own observations and the work of others in the field, we adapted the chronic stimulator implant technique for the treatment of facial anesthesia dolorosa in 1971. For our procedure, multicontact electrodes are implanted stereotactically using anatomical and electrophysiological parameters to determine the precise loci for implantation. The multicontact electrode is an extremely flexible cable composed of seven intertwined, separately insulated, platinum-iridium strands, each of which ter-

---

[1] The author wishes to acknowledge the support of the Lorenzo Lo Pain fund.

minates in a separate contact region spaced 2 mm apart on the cable axis. Each contact region is formed by wrapping an insulation-free strand end several times around the cable shaft. The diameter of the shaft is approximately 0.3 mm; the contact is approximately 0.5 mm in diameter and 0.5 mm long, with an effective surface area of 1.5 mm^2.

Initially, the electrodes are externalized for a temporary trial stimulation period that ranges from a few weeks to several months. If electrical stimulation of the brain proves to control the patient's pain satisfactorily during this trial period, then the electrodes are permanently implanted and connected internally to a subcutaneous radio frequency-coupled receiving unit for transcutaneous stimulation patterns.

Encouraged by the initial successful results of this procedure, we began to explore the possibility of using the technique for the treatment of other deafferentation pain or central pain syndromes. We soon found that chronic stimulation of the sensory nucleus of the thalamus was primarily useful in treating facial anesthesia dolorosa and trigeminal postherpetic neuralgia [1], and that stimulation of the posterior limb of the internal capsule at the posterior commissure level produced persistent relief from the discomforts of the thalamic syndrome, paraplegic pain, and phantom limb pain – with varying degrees of success. The majority of our patients who suffered the thalamic syndrome (8 out of 10) responded well to chronic stimulation of the posterior limb of the internal capsule, although satisfactory pain relief seemed to depend upon the size of the initial infarction [1]. However, patients whose pain was caused by the lateral medullary syndrome and by postcordotomy dysesthesia did not respond to stimulation of either the internal capsule or the sensory thalamic nucleus on a long-term basis [1].

ANDERSON et al. [3] investigated the cause of facial paresthesia following retrogasserian rhizotomy in cats. By monitoring the deafferented spinal trigeminal nucleus and making serial microelectrode recordings of neuronal activity in the feline brain stem, they found that spontaneous neuronal hyperactivity occurred 8–10 days following rhizotomy, and increased to a peak level 1 month after the operation. They postulated that this deafferentation-induced hyperactivity is a physiological correlate of the paresthesia experienced by patients after sectioning of the trigeminal nerve root.

In ANDERSON's study, the animals that experienced thalamic stimulation by means of implanted thalamic electrodes exhibited the appropriate short latency responses in the spinal trigeminal nucleus on the deafferentated side, as well as on the intact side. However, the cells within the deafferentated trigeminal complex that responded to thalamic stimulation did not exhibit spontaneous hyperactivity. The authors therefore suggested that the cells that responded to antidromic thalamic stimulation were interneurons that had not been directly deafferentated by rhizotomy. Since the effect of thalamic stimulation on neuronal hyperactivity was not demonstrated in this study, the results neither support nor refute our findings with PVM stimulation for the treatment of facial anesthesia dolorosa and trigeminal postherpetic neuralgia.

It is possible that the mechanism by which PVM stimulation acts to control pain may operate at the thalamic level also. The work of ZORUB and RICHARDSON [14] suggests that stimulation of the PVL-PVM complex may exert an inhibitory effect on the centrum medianum/parafascicular complex, where 'protopathic' sensation is thought to terminate.

Deductions concerning the precise neurophysiological substratum that responds to stimulation of the posterior limb of the internal capsule, and ameliorates the thalamic syndrome and phantom limb pain, are based on empirical results that do not yet present a unified theory of the origin of pain. The observed analgesic effects could be due to the activation of cortical inhibitory cells, as proposed by MOUNTCASTLE and POWELL [8], or to the augmentation of the descending control system, as suggested by ALBE-FESSARD et al. [2] and her colleagues, as well as by FETZ [4]. It is interesting that some patients with the thalamic syndrome have reported that their handwriting, ability to experience sensation, and coordination of the involved limbs have improved subsequent to internal capsule stimulation. Upon stimulation, patients have shown marked improvement in two-point discrimination and stereognosis, as well as a *decreased* acute pain threshold, as tested by a radiant-heat dolorimeter [5]. Whether or not these epiphenomena represent sensory augmentation secondary to facilitation of the corticothalamic reverberating circuit is purely conjectural.

In addition to the sensory thalamic nuclei and the internal capsule, a third locus of the brain recently has been recognized as a potential site for achieving pain control using the electrical stimulation technique. Since REYNOLDS [10] first reported that abdominal surgery could be performed without apparent discomfort during electrical stimulation of the midbrain, central, or periaqueductal gray matter in the unanesthetized rat, the literature has rapidly reinforced his observation. The efficacy of stimulation-produced analgesia has been demonstrated in the cat and monkey, as well as in the rat, and RICHARDSON and AKIL [11] now report that chronic, clinical pain states, as well as normal pain appreciation, can be blocked with the use of electrical stimulation in homologous medial brain stem regions in man.

Since these regions involve the seratogenic bulbospinal system, their results indicate that electrical stimulation can induce powerful, descending presynaptic inhibition at the dorsal horn level, and affect the central transmission of nociceptive information. We have implanted electrodes for long-term stimulation therapy in 3 of our patients suffering from the pain of disseminated cancer. The initial analgesic effect induced by electrical stimulation of the periaqueductal gray matter is astounding, although it becomes less effective over a period of a few months. Our observations suggest that continued stimulation may produce a chronic depletion of transmitter substance in the bulbospinal system [9]. There are indications that this process may be reversed by abstinence from stimulation.

In our experience with the use of brain stimulation for pain control in the sensory nuclei of the thalamus, the internal capsule, and the periaqueductal gray matter, we have observed practically no complications or side effects in our patients [6]. Our observations currently suggest that sensory thalamus and internal capsule stimulation is most efficacious for the control of various kinds of CNS pain, and that periaqueductal gray stimulation is appropriate for controlling pain of peripheral origin. Despite the need for more extensive neuroanatomical and neurophysiological studies in this area, there is now reason to hope that a nondestructive, nonaddictive means of alleviating chronic pain will soon be found.

References

1. ADAMS, J.E.; HOSOBUCHI, Y., and LINCHITZ, R.: The present status of implantable intracranial stimulators for pain. Clin. Neurosurg. *24* ch. 26, 347–361 (1977).
2. ALBE-FESSARD, D.; BESSON, J.M.; GUILBAUD, G., and LEVANTE, A.: Cortical control of somatic inflow into medial thalamus; in FRIGYESI, RINVIK and YAHS Cortico-thalamic projections and sensorimotor activities, pp. 283–303 (Raven Press, New York 1972).
3. ANDERSON, L.S.; BLACK, R.G.; ABRAHAM, J., and WARD, A.A., Jr.: Neuronal hyperactivity in experimental trigeminal deafferentation. J. Neurosurg. *35:* 444–452 (1971).
4. FETZ, E.E.: Pyramidal tract effects in the cat lumbar dorsal horn. J. Neurophysiol. *31:* 69–80 (1968).
5. HOSOBUCHI, Y.: Sensory threshold study during internal capsule stimulations. Read before the 1st World Congress on Pain, Florence 1975.
6. HOSOBUCHI, Y.; ADAMS, J.E., and LINCHITZ, R.: Pain relief by electrical stimulation of the central gray matter in humans and its reversal by naloxone. Science *197:* 183–186 (1977).
7. HOSOBUCHI, Y,; ADAMS, J.E., and RUTKIN, B.: Chronic thalamic stimulation for the control of facial anesthesia dolorosa. Archs. Neurol. *29:* 158–161 (1973).

8   Mountcastle, V.B. and Powell, T.P.S.: Neural mechanisms subserving cutaneous sensibility with special reference to the role of afferent inhibition in sensory perception and discrimination. Bull. Johns Hopkins Hosp. *105:* 201–232 (1959).
9   Oliveras, J.L.; Hosobuchi, Y.; Gilbaud, G., and Besson, J.M.: Analgesic electrical stimulation of the central gray matter in cats and its reversal by 5-HTP. Brain Res. (in press).
10 Reynolds, D.V.: Surgery in the rat during electrical analgesia induced by focal brain stimulation. Science *164:* 444–445 (1969).
11 Richardson, D.E. and Akil, H.: Pain reduction by electrical brain stimulation in man. J. Neurosurg. *47:* 184–194 (1977).
12 Shealy, C.N.; Mortimer, J.T., and Hagfors, N.R.: Dorsal column electroanalgesia. J. Neurosurg. *32:* 560–564 (1970).
13 White, J.C. and Sweet, W.H.: Pain and the neurosurgeon. A 40-year experience, p. 218 (Thomas, Springfield 1969).
14 Zorub, D.S. and Richardson, D.F.: Thalamic projection of the extralemniscal sensory system. Read before the American Association of Neurological Surgeons, Houston 1971.

Dr. Yoshio Hosobuchi, Associate Professor of Neurosurgery, University of California School of Medicine, *San Francisco, CA* 94122 (USA)